D0374501

HEALTH CARE

HEALTH CARE

Pat Armstrong and Hugh Armstrong

About Canada Series

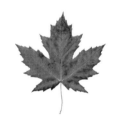

Fernwood Publishing • Halifax & Winnipeg

Copyright © 2008 Pat Armstrong and Hugh Armstrong

All rights reserved. No part of this book may be reproduced or transmitted in any form by any means without permission in writing from the publisher, except by a reviewer, who may quote brief passages in a review.

Editing: Robert Clarke
Cover Art: John van der Woude
Printed and bound in Canada by Hignell Book Printing
Printed on paper containing 100% post-consumer fibre.

Published in Canada by Fernwood Publishing
Site 2A, Box 5, 32 Oceanvista Lane
Black Point, Nova Scotia, B0J 1B0
and #8 - 222 Osborne Street, Winnipeg, Manitoba, R3L 1Z3
www.fernwoodpublishing.ca

Fernwood Publishing Company Limited gratefully acknowledges the financial support of the Government of Canada through the Book Publishing Industry Development Program (BPDIP), the Canada Council for the Arts and the Nova Scotia Department of Tourism and Culture for our publishing program.

 Canadian Heritage Patrimoine canadien   The Canada Council for the Arts Le Conseil des Arts du Canada   NOVA SCOTIA Tourism and Culture

Library and Archives Canada Cataloguing in Publication

Armstrong, Pat, 1945-
Health care / Pat Armstong and Hugh Armstrong.

(About Canada)
Includes bibliographical references.
ISBN 978-1-55266-246-5

1. Medical care–Canada. 2. Medical policy–Canada. 3. Public health–Canada. I. Armstrong, Hugh, 1943- II. Title. III. Series: About Canada (Black Point, N.S.)

RA395.C3A74 2008   362.10971   C2007-903360-1

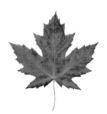

CONTENTS

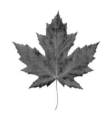

1. WHY CARE?

Our public system of health care is in trouble. These days it seems we can't watch television, listen to the radio, log onto the Internet, or read a newspaper or magazine without encountering some horror story. This week comes news of a cancer patient in desperate need of a drug not recognized or covered by the public system. Last week it was an elderly woman who couldn't find a doctor, and the week before that an elderly man had to wait a year for hip surgery. The week before that it was an athlete with torn ligaments who couldn't get an MRI. Tomorrow it might be an infection acquired in the hospital by a new mother. Next week it might be someone who can't get an appointment with a specialist.

Even the Supreme Court of Canada has entered the fray. In 2004, in what became widely known as the Chaoulli case, the Court agreed to hear a case about the alleged failure of the public health system—what we call medicare. It heard experts testifying about major shortages in the public system. Four out of the seven presiding judges concluded that the system was indeed in trouble, at least in Quebec.

While we hear story after story about how the system fails individuals, we are increasingly warned that worse is yet to come. All those babies born after World War II, when the soldiers came home and prosperity returned, are growing old. These aging baby boomers, we are told, will put heavy pressure on the public health-care system, risking bankruptcy for us all. Not only are there a lot of them, but they are also likely to live longer than the previous generation. Moreover, new technologies and drugs come at ever higher prices—prices that the public purse will not be able to handle. Radio, television, magazines, and the Internet carry constant talk about new pandemics, while a lot of noisy advertising tells us about yet another worrisome health problem coming our way.

For some time now, given this barrage of bad news, Canadians have been expressing concern, even panic, about their public health-care system. Indeed, "be scared" seems to be the message. The personal stories bring the problems home, suggesting, "This could be me." The constant weight of all these stories—and especially the threat of too many old people, combined with more expensive drugs and more illness—suggests that the public system is no longer sustainable, that public care is a luxury we can no longer afford. The need to do something seems to be increasingly urgent.

What is this public system that's in the news so much? At its core, medicare covers the costs of much of our health care when we need it, and it does so without direct charge. We don't person-ally pay the hospital or the doctor that provides us with care. As a result, financial barriers almost never prevent us from seeking care for ourselves or our family members. Instead, the costs are met by governments—we pay through our taxes. As a society we pool the risk of encountering ill health, which means that the healthy and wealthy foot most of the bill, rather than the unhealthy and poor. It also means that some of the healthy and wealthy want to reduce or even eliminate this pooling of health risks, and their voices are often powerful. *Pool health risks.*

Despite this power, and despite all the turmoil surrounding it, medicare remains Canada's best-loved social program. For many people it is also a defining feature of our country. It represents our commitment to shared responsibility and our recognition of shared vulnerability. Losing it would mean much more than losing access to care; it would mean losing a symbol that is the essence of the

Canada that emerged from World War II committed to democratic and solidaristic means of achieving our right to care. Still, we are right to be afraid, although not necessarily for the reasons given in the stories.

Canadians are being offered a variety of solutions to these troubles, all of them advertised as saving public care. But to assess these solutions, we must dig more deeply into the past, present, and possible future makeup of the system. We need to find out what the evidence tells us about what works for whom, along with who benefits most from the solutions being offered. We need to examine the claims that the system is now in crisis, rather than assuming that this is the case. Given that we have a public health-care system, we all have a stake in the system. It belongs to us, and it is up to us to determine its future. We can do this only if we know what we have—including where it has come from—as well as what we don't have. We need to look at what we need, what we could have, and what we could lose if we let it all somehow drift away.

We need, too, to look more closely at the manufacturing of dissent on the health-care front, and especially at the possible solutions being put forward: private insurance and the right to buy care, along with for-profit delivery and management. As we shall see, the evidence does not support these forms of privatization as viable solutions. Instead, we need strategies developed through the public system to further improve quality, access, efficiency, and equity. In other words, we need collective, democratic strategies for care. We need these strategies not only to protect health care but also to protect our understanding of Canada as a place that puts shared solutions above the individual's right to buy and profit from care.

Like the United Nations, the authors of this book see health care as a human right, which means that necessary health-care services should not be a source of profit. This is not just our opinion. As Roy Romanow, who headed the Commission on the Future of Health Care, put it in 2002 after examining the evidence and consulting Canadians widely, health care is about our values and it is as sustainable as we collectively want it to be. He called his report *Building on Values*, emphasizing the centrality of values in seeking solutions. Our health-care system is fundamentally about democracy, and democracy can work only with a public that is both involved and informed. It will also work only if those who participate in the debate make their values explicit. We intend this book to contribute to the democratic process by offering the tools needed for informed involvement in the shaping of public care.

The evidence and the values of most Canadians are both on the side of keeping medicare public; indeed, they are both on the side of expanding its public scope and character. But the powerful forces favouring privatization are not disappearing quietly into the night. They keep finding new ways of promoting their interests. To defend and to improve our public system require at least as much vigilance on our side. This book is intended as a contribution to the democratic and continuing fight on behalf of medicare.

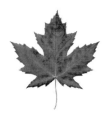

2. HOW DID WE GET HERE?

"My name is Sally. I work in intensive care, and I'm benefited," a California nurse told us in the late 1990s when asked to describe her job. We were doing group interviews with nurses in the United States, and nurse after nurse said much the same thing. Although we had been interviewing Canadian nurses for years, that was the first time we heard the term "benefited"—and for good reason, as it turns out. What this California nurse meant was that, in her job, she had health insurance. In a country in which health-care costs are the leading cause of personal bankruptcy, and where most of the people who have health insurance get it through employment, the matter of "benefits" is among the first questions asked by people seeking a job. And "benefits" mean, above all, health insurance in various forms.

In Canada health-care coverage is not tied to employment, and few health-sector workers would describe their work in terms of health benefits. Indeed, many of the Canadians we have interviewed have no idea what is covered under their supplementary health

> "Critics of government-run health care are either rich hypochondriacs who want to buy more medical services than the state will allow them, or lousy economists."
>
> —Columnist Eric Reguly, *Globe and Mail Report on Business*, February 6, 1999, p. B2.

plan, when they do have one. After close to fifty years of public care Canadians take basic coverage for granted, even in the face of the growing panic. How did we get a public health-care system while the richest nation in the world leaves more than forty-seven million people without health-care coverage, and many more with inadequate coverage? To understand our quite different trajectories, we have to look back as far as the early part of the twentieth century.

Depressions and Wars, Economics and Ideas

The Great Depression and World War II were both critical to the introduction of public health care in Canada. The stock market crashed in 1929, signalling the failure of free-market capitalism. Governments across Canada responded to the subsequent dramatic rise in unemployment by following classical economic theories that said, "Leave the market alone." Governments provided a modicum of public relief for people who were defined as the most deserving and vulnerable. Widows with children were most likely to receive this charity, although it was dependent upon the close inspection of their lives. Others were eligible for workfare—very low-wage, back-breaking labour that went mainly to men deemed employable. Many were left to ride the rails in search of employment or to beg from door to door for food. Protests were inevitable, and were just as inevitably put down. People paid their doctors and hospitals in food and services, or not at all. Many simply went without care.

As the Depression both continued and deepened, governments began to listen to a new theory being put forward by a British economist, John Maynard Keynes. Simply put, he challenged two supposedly common-sense notions. The first is that governments should not interfere in the marketplace, leaving the economy instead to business to run. The second is that governments should stop spending when their supply of money is low. Instead, Keynes argued that governments should spend in bad times, creating demand for both employees and products. They should borrow in order to purchase public goods like roads, schools, and hospitals, and they should put money into the hands of the unemployed. In good times governments should save in ways that would allow them to protect workers and their purchasing power from excessive inflation. With money to spend even when they are unemployed, people would sustain the demand for goods and services and thus promote employment. Keynes also argued that a healthy, skilled labour force was both critical to the economy and a government responsibility. Many Canadian policy analysts —most notably social scientist Leonard Marsh[1]—promoted similar ideas and even more government-sponsored programs to support a healthy, educated labour force.

World War II reinforced Keynes's views. When Canada entered the war in 1939, governments were not in good economic shape. Nevertheless, they invested heavily in everything from guns to day care. Employment and training expanded enormously, including in the health-care sector, where large numbers of women found work. Recruitment and conscription brought many people directly into government service. However, a health survey found that too many Canadians did not make the grade for entry into military service, laying the groundwork for future government intervention in health issues. War also meant heavy investment in the development of new drugs, technologies, and techniques to deal with the casualties. Some of these, like antibiotics and plastic surgery, transformed treatments, while the recruitment of so many workers transformed care. Together these developments in health services contributed to the need for large hospitals where the complex equipment could most efficiently be utilized.

The sacrifices of war were promoted on the grounds of solidarity with Britain, the protection of freedom, and the promise of a better world to come. The war itself encouraged feelings and programs of solidarity, bringing people together through both deprivation and action. Countries such as Canada and the United States emerged from World War II with a commitment not only to peace and prosperity but also to human rights. Indeed, a Canadian official took the lead in drafting an international declaration of human rights at the United Nations. Increasingly, shared responsibility for what were understood as shared risks was a notion that underlined Canadian government activities, rather than the idea that most people got what they deserved in a market economy and must be held responsible for themselves.

The legacy of the war was a significantly expanded state, a sense of common cause, and expectations of government intervention to both provide and protect. The war also left a significant proportion of the population with military experience, creating the possibility of a formidable opposition. Governments remembered the major protests that followed World War I, and feared a repeat. Unions and women's groups, religious organizations, and community groups became increasingly active in demanding public health care. Governments were already heavily involved in providing health services for the military and for veterans. Services for those who had sacrificed at home seemed a logical extension.

The end of World War II also signalled the return of economic prosperity, thanks in large measure to government intervention. Governments had spent a great deal on the goods and services needed to fight the war, in the process reviving many businesses that had failed during the Depression. Governments also limited the right to buy during the war in order to save materials and labour for the war effort. When the war ended, they continued to spend on housing, health care, and education for returning veterans. As a result, there was lots of pent-up demand for houses, cars, furniture, and frivolity as well as lots of money to buy them with, thanks to forced wartime saving and rising postwar employment. Although governments still had debts from the war, prosperity meant that rising tax revenues went along with the increases in employment levels.

Politics and People

It took more than popular demand and good economic times, new economic theories and the positive experience of government intervention to get public care. It also took political will on the part of both individuals and governments. The most famous of these individuals was Tommy Douglas. He may be the grandfather of the popular TV and movie actor Keifer Sutherland, but years after his death Douglas remains justly famous in his own right. In 2005 he was voted the greatest Canadian ever in a major CBC television program poll.

Tommy Douglas had an infection in his leg when he was young, and he would have lost that leg if he had been forced to depend on his family's ability to pay for care. His family had no insurance, and it was only by accident that a doctor decided to offer his services while using the boy to demonstrate a technique that saved his leg. Douglas vowed then to work hard to ensure that no one's health depended on charity and accident. Unlike most of us who make pledges in our youth, he followed through on his when he became premier of Saskatchewan in 1944. Even though Saskatchewan was heavily in debt and one of the poorest provinces, he carried out his promise. In 1947, just two years after the end of World War II, his social-democratic government introduced the first public hospital insurance plan in Canada. This plan became the model for our public health-care system and a key element in his vision of a better, fairer Saskatchewan and Canada.

The hospital insurance plan certainly had its opponents, with many critics expressing fear about government intervention and the loss of private control. At the time, however, hospitals in Canada were almost all owned and operated by non-profit charitable or religious organizations. Many of them were in deep financial trouble because so many patients could not pay for hospital services. To survive they needed government money, though they also wanted to remain independent. When patients did have insurance, it was mainly from non-profit organizations, such as Blue Cross, formed by hospitals themselves. So these insurance companies were protecting hospitals, not profits. Employees of the hospitals were supportive. They had an interest in stable government funding, rather than uncertain insurance-based support. In any case, most of the employees were low-paid women who were not then represented by unions and thus were not very influential in the decision-making process. Employers outside health care were starting to face unions that were demanding that they provide hospital insurance, so they too were not strongly opposed to some government payment. A public plan means costs are shared across the population, relieving pressure on employers to pay.

What the Saskatchewan government under Douglas offered was a public insurance plan that covered everyone in the province. Payment came from taxes while the hospitals were left mainly to run themselves. Those who could, paid premiums. But the same hospital care was available to all, regardless of ability to pay.

Douglas was successful in part because we have a parliamentary system of government. In Canada the party with the majority forms the government. Given that governments can be forced out of office if they lose a vote, strong party discipline pushes all members of the governing party to support the government in a vote. This in turn makes it harder for opponents of a measure to influence votes by influencing individual members of parliament.

This political system contrasts with the United States. As anyone who watched the U.S. TV show *The West Wing* knows, individual members of Congress can be pressured by companies and organizations opposed to a piece of legislation to vote against it without threatening their party. Private interests thus have more direct power. Even a president with a majority in Congress can therefore find it difficult to pass health-care legislation, as Bill Clinton found in the early 1990s when he was president.

Douglas's plan for Saskatchewan was a success. Even those who had initially opposed the plan came to see the benefits of a program that not only allowed everyone who needed hospital care to get it but also ensured that hospitals were paid. In the years that followed the government did not go broke, as some had predicted, and patients received good care, contrary to other predictions. As more and more people saw that the plan worked, more and more of them supported it. In other words, the success created support. And success often breeds imitation.

Other provinces, and their populations, saw the plan working. So too did the federal government. As a result, growing demands came from individuals, organizations, and regional governments to follow in Saskatchewan's footsteps. Attempts to get a public scheme across Canada were not new, but earlier attempts had hit the same wall that we come up against too often today: namely, resistance from the provinces based on the fear of federal government interference in provincial territory. According to the *British North America Act*, the constitution that governed Canada until replaced by the *Canada Act in 1982*, health care is primarily a provincial responsibility. When the federal government tried to set a national health-care plan in place right after World War II, the provinces would not agree and the attempt failed. Foiled in its efforts to organize health-care services, the federal government responded by offering funds for hospital construction and the education of health-care personnel. This funding contributed to the enormous expansion of hospitals but left the provinces, insurance companies, and individuals with the bills for services. This, in turn, led to more provincial governments seeking federal financial help.

The small provinces, and the poorer ones, were interested in a more comprehensive federal plan, but the big, rich provinces continued to resist. Sound familiar? It should, because the same scenario is played out today every time the federal government seeks to introduce new programs. In the 1950s, though, instead of giving in to Ontario, Quebec, Alberta, and British Columbia, the federal government introduced a plan anyway. In 1957 it passed legislation introducing a national hospital insurance plan. It offered to pay half of all hospital operating costs if the provinces agreed to conform to certain basic principles. Take it or leave it was the offer. In the end it was an offer no province could refuse. It took political will on the part of the federal government to make this plan happen and, when it did, the program was a great success. Like the Saskatchewan plan, the federal scheme built support through its success.

Our system began, then, with a war and with a province and with dedicated and determined individuals, backed by efforts from organized groups within the union movement, the faith community, social welfare policy circles, and elsewhere to bring about change that would benefit us all. It also began with hospitals, an approach that in itself became a critical legacy.

Doctors and Evidence

While the new plan paid for hospitals, most doctors were not part of the program—so that is where, in the late 1950s, Douglas in Saskatchewan next moved. He proposed to have the doctors paid salaries by the government, a step taken in the United Kingdom soon after World War II. But Douglas would face much fiercer opposition this time around.

During the Great Depression of the 1930s, many doctors in Saskatchewan and elsewhere in the country had supported the idea of more government involvement in the payment for care. Not just during the Depression but also in previous years, doctors had often gone without payment. Some had become involved in setting up non-profit insurance plans to cover physician care, but this still left many patients without either insurance or the means to pay for care. Many doctors, like many other Canadians, also supported more public health care as a way of ensuring a human right.

By the time Saskatchewan tried to introduce an insurance plan to cover doctors, postwar prosperity had returned and more patients could afford to pay. At the same time the rise of the Soviet Union and the beginning of the Cold War made many in the West more suspicious of government intervention. Doctors, with their long tradition of private, independent practice, worried about interference with their incomes and ways of providing care. As well, more private, for-profit insurance companies were involved in this field, and they too resisted government insurance schemes.

As a result, doctors organized their own resistance to the Saskatchewan proposal for the introduction of public medical insurance and to the idea that they be placed on salary. They also organized many of their patients, suggesting that the outcome of the government scheme would be a loss not only of doctors but also of privacy and choice. Most of the doctors even went on strike, although many doctors supported the Saskatchewan government plan and continued to work. With considerable support from community organizations and unions, the majority social-democratic government responded both by bringing in doctors from the United Kingdom—doctors who supported public health care—and by modifying its proposal.

In the end Saskatchewan did for the doctors what it had done for hospitals. The 1962 legislation left doctors largely alone to practise as they had been doing and organized an insurance scheme to pay for their services. Instead of becoming salaried employees, doctors continued in private practice, but with their fees paid by the government. The fees were negotiated with the government by the doctors' professional organization. As David Naylor, president of the University of Toronto, puts it in his book on the growth of doctors' power, it was public payment for private practice, with everyone covered for doctor care.[2]

Once again the scheme worked, and its success worked to build further support. Once again Saskatchewan served as a model for the federal government. This time, however, the federal government under Progressive Conservative prime minister John Diefenbaker was more cautious. It gave in to demands from doctors and established a Royal Commission to investigate alternatives, with Supreme Court Justice Emmett Hall as its head. Significantly, Justice Hall did not begin as a supporter of a universal public scheme. He was pressured by many individual doctors and by the Canadian Medical Association to recommend a plan that would have the government pay for the poor, the elderly, the disabled, and the military, but would leave everyone else to pay for their own care. The evidence presented to Hall, however, convinced him that a single system was the most efficient and effective. It would cost too much to sort the deserving from the undeserving, especially given that most people would be eligible for some form of economic support.

After a lengthy public consultation period and some primary research, the *Report of the Royal Commission on Health Services* (Hall Report 1964–65) recommended a single payment system that covered everyone for doctor care as part of a scheme including the full range of health services. The Commission argued that covering all services, from hospitals to long-term care and home care, from drugs to doctors, dentists and nurses, would ensure that the sick were cared for at the most appropriate level of care in ways that would increase efficiency and effectiveness. Otherwise, administrative costs would be too high and millions would be excluded. In addition to arguing for the inclusion of health services such as eye and dental care, ambulances, and nursing stations in the North, Hall argued for preventive programs such as water fluoridation, and for the preparation of more health-care providers.

The federal government under Liberal prime minister Lester Pearson took up immediately only the recommendation on doctors, and the *Medical Care Act* became law in 1966. The government intended to move on to other services later.

According to Dennis Gruending, Emmett Hall's biographer, "The doctors were stunned."[3] Over the next few years, as first the smaller, poorer provinces and then the larger, richer provinces considered whether to take up the federal offer of shared payment for universal access to medical services, the doctors organized resistance. In 1970, however, just as the larger provinces were reaching their decisions to join in, the doctors' protests were halted by a bigger crisis in Canada. A group supporting Quebec independence, the FLQ, kidnapped a British diplomat and later kidnapped and killed a provincial cabinet minister. It was difficult to hold demonstrations on Parliament Hill to oppose the federal government when others were there supporting that government. The doctors' protests fizzled, and all of the provinces ended up passing legislation agreeing to the federal scheme to provide universal insurance to cover physician care.

So What Else Is New?

Since that time, no new major health-care programs have been introduced at the federal level, despite the good intentions of various succeeding governments. Justice Hall was asked to look at the system again in 1979 by the Progressive Conservative government headed by Joe Clark. A couple of decades later, two further investigations on the future of health care were established by Liberal governments headed by Prime Minister Jean Chrétien. Like the second Hall Report (1980), the National Forum on Health (1997) and the Romanow Royal Commission on the Future of Health Care (2002) echoed the original Hall Report.[4] They all reviewed the available information and conducted new research. They also all concluded that Canada should expand the public system and keep it universal, because that is not only the most equitable but also the most efficient and effective approach. Although a Senate committee headed by Michael Kirby began by supporting more private payment, and even though it did not undertake the kind of systematic research or consultation that the other inquiries did, it too concluded in 2002 that a system of public payment was the preferred option.[5]

Even so, significant developments have taken place since medicare was first introduced. The federal government's promise to pay the provinces for half the costs of hospital and doctor care was changed in the wake of rising and not very predictable expenditures. Instead, in 1977 the federal government gave up some areas of taxation to the provinces, allowing them to raise the money directly, and it introduced a complex formula called Established Program Financing (EPF). Under EPF the reduced cash transfers were based on the number of people in each province and the rate of economic growth. A formula ensured that the poorer provinces were not disproportionately deprived by this new financial arrangement. The proportion of the health-care money coming directly from the federal government gradually began to decline, reaching about 15 percent of what the provinces spent, while the provinces retained the tax room or "points" obtained in 1977.

The decline accelerated as successive federal governments moved away from Keynesian economics and back to the old idea of a reliance on markets to meet all needs. This recycled approach

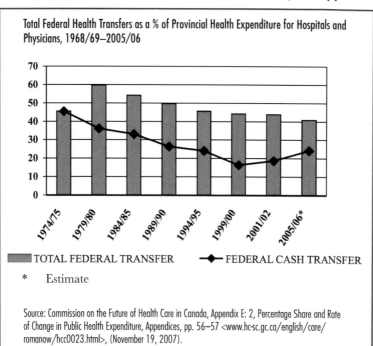

Total Federal Health Transfers as a % of Provincial Health Expenditure for Hospitals and Physicians, 1968/69–2005/06

TOTAL FEDERAL TRANSFER   ◆— FEDERAL CASH TRANSFER

* Estimate

Source: Commission on the Future of Health Care in Canada, Appendix E: 2, Percentage Share and Rate of Change in Public Health Expenditure, Appendices, pp. 56–57 <www.hc-sc.gc.ca/english/care/romanow/hcc0023.html>, (November 19, 2007).

not only rejected new government programs as inappropriate but also called for less government intervention in existing social policy fields. Those in favour of this approach promoted panic over the debt and deficit. Both social programs and dependent individuals were blamed for the crisis, even though research showed that the main causes of the federal government's debt were the cuts to taxes for corporations and rising interest charges.

Responding to international and national pressure, as well as to a shift among their own supporters, the federal government under both Progressive Conservatives (from 1984 to 1993) and Liberals (from 1993 to 2006) embraced this neo-liberal approach. Federal funding for health, education, and welfare dropped particularly drastically in 1996, when the federal government introduced yet another funding formula, the Canada Health and Social Transfer (CHST). The CHST rolled the funding for all three program areas into one package and reduced the funding by an amount equal to what had been previously going to welfare. In 2003 and again in 2004, as government coffers filled, as debts receded even with further tax cuts, and as public outcries against cuts to medicare increased, the federal government provided significant new money to the provinces and territories for health care. As part of a 2004 agreement between the federal and provincial/territorial governments, the federal government committed to transferring an additional $41 billion over ten years, bringing the direct federal share of provincial/territorial health spending back up to 25 percent.

The changes made before 2003 had effects beyond the deterioration in health services resulting directly from cuts in spending. Public confidence in and support for medicare suffered, and the federal government lost much of its leadership role. It was the prospect of federal transfer payments that enticed all the provinces to become part of the national program. It is the withdrawal of this money that is the stick to ensure that provinces conform to the principles and conditions set out by the federal government. By meeting less of the cost of provincial health services, and by unilaterally cutting the funds it did provide, the federal government lost leverage with the provinces. It now largely allows them to follow their own paths. The federal government also lost credibility with the public.

Cutbacks by successive governments demonstrated a reduced commitment to shared responsibility and reduced support for government involvement in social programs. The 2004 federal funding increase, and a major one at that, came with virtually no strings attached. Provinces and territories can spend the money on roads or tax cuts rather than on health care. Not surprisingly, given the horror stories and provincial practices, the funding increase failed to generate additional support for the Liberal government under Paul Martin, which lost the subsequent federal election. Meanwhile, the minority Conservative federal government elected in 2006 followed the policy of its predecessor in actively supporting more private profit in health care. Despite continuing popular support for medicare and promises to protect public care, the political will to expand national health-care programs has not been there. Little has happened to carry out the recommendations from the federal reports on expanded coverage for prescription drugs and home care in particular.

Canada and the United States: Public versus Private

There are, then, several reasons as to why Canada has a public health-care program and the United States does not. Both countries went through the Great Depression and World War II, although Canada was in that war much longer. Both emerged from the war with a strong sense of shared risk, and both supported some form of public health care. Indeed, the support for such a system may even have been stronger in the United States.[6]

Part of the explanation for the difference can be found in our parliamentary system, which makes it more difficult for wealthy interest groups to undermine public policy by pressuring individual legislators. Part comes from the very nature of our federal system, which allows one province to introduce programs that can become models for the others. Part also springs from a long tradition of social democracy within specific areas of the country, places where individuals such as Tommy Douglas could have a significant impact. Another part of our tradition that matters is the practice of establishing royal commissions that can assess the evidence and consult Canadians. Unions, women's groups, and community organizations played critical roles in the consultations undertaken by the Hall and Romanow commissions in particular.

Finally, part of the explanation for the difference between the Canadian and U.S. experiences can be found in what political scientist Carolyn Tuohy calls accidental logics.[7] Both countries adopted incremental approaches to the development of comprehensive programs. Canada started with hospital construction, followed by hospital services and then doctor services. The United States focused on particular population groups: the poor, the elderly, the disabled, and the military. One unintended consequence of the U.S. system has been the politics of resentment. Wealthier people in both countries often resent paying through taxes for care that goes only to others. In Canada, rich and poor alike usually receive similar care, however expensive, so long as the care is deemed medically necessary. In the United States, even unions, once they have won health-care insurance at the bargaining table, have at times been at best tepid in their support for a public system.

It was clear from the first Hall Commission that a universal program is administratively cheaper. Very little time and thus money are spent sorting out the eligible from the ineligible for the single package of services available to all people who have the right to live in the country. Moreover, health-care providers don't have to set up elaborate systems to seek and negotiate payment from a bewildering array of funding sources. Our main unintended consequence has been the politics of solidarity. Those establishing medicare had little idea that it would become not only Canada's best-loved social program but also a defining feature of being Canadian.

The evidence is still overwhelmingly in favour of a public

health system. Once again, however, the country is seeing strong opposition from a vocal group of doctors and other critics who ignore this evidence. They are supported by very strong for-profit insurance companies and health-service organizations that were not particularly prominent in earlier times. Supporting the evidence are a majority of Canadians and those large corporations perceptive enough to recognize that a public health-care system gives them a competitive advantage because they don't have to pay for most of the health care of their current and former employees.

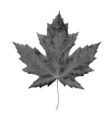

3. WHAT DID WE GET?

Another critical development occurred in the late 1970s after the introduction of national hospital and doctor insurance, paid for from tax revenues. This change too was shaped by a feisty individual and a royal commission, as well as by advocates and resisters, political philosophies, and economic times. As the initial policy of paying for half of provincial expenses was replaced with a funding formula that made expenditures more difficult to track and penalties more difficult to impose, advocates of public health came together in the Canadian Health Coalition in 1979 to warn that public care was under threat. A growing number of doctors were charging patients extra fees for their services. At the same time it was alleged that provincial governments were spending their health-care dollars on other things such as roads, schools, and tax cuts.

A second royal commission, again under Emmett Hall, was the response. Justice Hall concluded in 1980 that the fees were threatening accessibility to health services and the universality of the health plan. The federal minister of health, Monique Bégin, decided to take the doctors and the provinces on. Supported by labour unions, nurses, and health advocates, she convinced the Trudeau government that new legislation was required to make the rules clear. In late 1983 the federal government introduced what is probably our most famous piece of legislation, the *Canada Health Act*.

The *Canada Health Act*

The *Canada Health Act* is a remarkable piece of legislation. For one thing, it represented a clear defeat of strong physician opposition. Even a twenty-three-day doctor strike in Ontario in 1986 did not prevent the province from agreeing to its provisions when it became clear that the federal health minister would withhold funds if the provisions were violated. For another, it is very short for a document that has had such a lasting and profound impact since coming into law in 1984. At only thirteen pages, in both official languages, it sets out the principles and conditions that guide the health plans of our ten provinces and three territories, spread across a country with the second-largest land mass in the world. Contrast this with the thousands of pages in the plan that Hillary Clinton proposed for the United States in the early 1990s.

The act's length is, to a large extent, its strength. It made clear that we Canadians share common values when it comes to health care, while it allowed each province and territory to meet these principles and conditions in its own ways to meet its own needs and preferences. It consolidated and clarified the earlier hospital and doctor insurance bills, making the principles and conditions for federal funding explicit and simple.

The Famous Five

What have come to be known as the five principles of the *Canada Health Act* are the criteria that provinces and territories must meet in order to qualify for federal funding.

First, in importance at least, is universality. Everyone legally in the province, except tourists, visitors, and transients, must be covered for public health insurance under the same terms and conditions. It is a program that defines care as a right. It is this criterion that is central to the popularity of the plan and to the promotion of solidarity among Canadians.

Second is accessibility. To be accessible, services must be similar for everyone. This means that you cannot have some hospitals for the poor and others for the rich; some doctors for the poor and others for the rich. Health services must also be without financial or other barriers. Doctors are prohibited from extra-billing, from imposing charges on patients that are in addition to the fees the doctors receive from their provincial health insurance plan. Hospitals are likewise prohibited from imposing user fees, or charges to patients for essential services. At the same time, the act specifies that health professionals and hospitals must be reasonably compensated for their services. The accessibility criterion not only helps make universality real, but also reduces administrative costs for collecting fees. Research conducted in Quebec soon after medicare was introduced showed that the plan significantly improved access for those who needed care, and many of these people were poor.[1] Moreover, with everyone using the same services, everyone has a vested interest in ensuring that these services are effective.

A third criterion is comprehensiveness—a term that refers in this context to medical practitioners, to dentists performing required services in hospitals, and to hospitals, but not to all health services. Some provincial plans make provision for other providers to be covered, but it is not clear exactly what comprehensiveness means in practice. In general, the act provides very few details, preferring to leave a great deal up to the provinces in meeting this criterion. However, it does specify what is included in comprehensive hospital services. Accommodation and food are included. So too are all required drugs, tests and their interpretation, facilities, supplies, therapies, nursing, and any other services provided by people paid by the hospital. Even private rooms are listed, if they are medically required. In short, everything you need for care must be provided without charge while you are in the hospital. This too eliminates the need for expensive recording of each billable item. Meanwhile, there is no detailed definition of doctor care. Doctors themselves get to define what is medically necessary.

The fourth criterion, portability, also contributes directly both

Canada Health Act

Some excerpts:

Public Administration

(a) the health insurance plan of a province must be administered and operated on a non-profit basis by a public authority appointed or designated by the government of the province;

(b) the public authority must be responsible to the provincial government for that administration and operation; and

(c) the public authority must be subject to audit of its accounts and financial transactions by such authority as is charged by law with the audit of the accounts of the province.

Comprehensiveness

The health care insurance plan of a province must insure all insured health services provided by hospitals, medical practitioners or dentists, and where the law of the province so permits, similar or additional services rendered by other health care practitioners.

Universality

The health insurance plan of a province must entitle one hundred per cent of the insured persons of the province to the insured health services provided for by the plan on uniform terms and conditions.

Portability

The health care insurance plan of a province

(a) must not impose any minimum period of residence in the province, or waiting period, in excess of three months before residents of the province are eligible for or entitled to insured health services;

(b) must provide for and be administered and operated so as to provide for the payment of amounts for the cost of insured health services provided to insured persons while temporarily absent from the province on the basis that

(i) where the insured health services are provided in Canada, payment for health services is at the rate that is approved by the health care insurance plan of the province in which the services are provided, unless the provinces concerned agree to apportion the cost between them in a different manner, or

(ii) where the insured health services are provided out of Canada, payment is made on the basis of the amount that would have been paid by the province for similar services rendered in the province, with due regard, in the case of hospital services, to the size of the hospital, standards of service and other relevant factors; and

(c) must provide for and be administered and operated so as to provide for the payment, during any minimum period of residence, or any waiting period, imposed by the health care insurance plan of another province, of the cost of insured services provided to persons who have ceased to be insured persons of that other province, on the same basis as though they had not ceased to be residents of the province.

Accessibility

The health care insurance plan of a province

(a) must provide for insured health services on uniform terms and conditions and on a basis that does not impede or preclude, either directly or indirectly whether by charges made to the insured persons or otherwise, reasonable access to those services by insured person;

(b) must provide for payment for insured services in accordance with a tariff or system of payment authorized by the law of the province;

(c) must provide for reasonable compensation for all insured health services rendered by medical practitioners or dentists; and

(d) must provide for the payment of amounts to hospitals, including hospitals owned or operated by Canada, in respect of the cost of insured health services.

to the efficiency of the system and to universality. You can take health insurance with you from province to province in Canada. If you are visiting another province and get sick or injured, your home province must pay for the needed care, and pay at the going rate for the province where the care is provided. If you move to another province, you take your health insurance with you for three months until you are covered by the province to which you moved. If you need some complicated procedure, such as an organ transplant, but the procedure is not performed in, say, Prince Edward Island, where you live, you may with the prior approval of your province have it performed in, say, Nova Scotia, with payment made by the province you live in.

That is what the act says about portability, but our health care is also portable in two other senses. Unlike most people in the United States, Canadians can take our health care from job to job. And unlike many U.S. citizens who rely on private insurance, we can also take our care from service to service, with the right to choose which service we use. In the Russell Crowe movie *The Insider*, for example, the father, working in the United States, felt he could not leave his job at a tobacco company even when he found its behaviour immoral, and that was because his asthmatic daughter would lose her health-care coverage. In Canada we are signed up to a provincial or territorial plan that allows us to carry our insurance with us throughout the system, regardless of our location or employment. This feature allows Canadians far more choice than our U.S. counterparts enjoy; choice in jobs, in doctors, and in hospitals.

Finally, the act requires that the health insurance plan of each province or territory be publicly administered. This means that the insurance plan is administered by a non-profit agency that is responsible to the government and is subject to audit. This criterion creates at least the possibility of democratic control and scrutiny.

The two conditions set out in the *Canada Health Act* are quite simple. Provinces must report to the federal government each year on how they are meeting the five criteria or principles, and they must acknowledge the financial contribution from the federal government.

Why Is Medicare a Symbol of Canada?

> Canadians embrace medicare as a public good, a national symbol and a defining aspect of their citizenship.
>
> Source: Roy Romanow, *Building on Values*, p. xviii.

What we got with the *Canada Health Act*—our basic medicare system —was a symbol of Canada, a key element distinguishing us from the United States. It is a symbol implying that we care for each other. It recognizes that we have a shared responsibility as well as a shared risk of ill health. It symbolizes a commitment to health care as a human right, open to all. It is a symbol for good reasons, one of which is that it has indeed provided reasonable access to care. Not only that, but it is also by most measures uniformly good care. Access has become significantly more equitable not only for the rich and poor but also among the provinces as extra federal funds support care in jurisdictions that lack the resources to provide reasonable access on their own. A U.S. doctor told us that the first test done in his hospital is a "wallet biopsy." With public insurance for doctor and hospital care, this is an unknown procedure in Canadian hospitals and doctors' offices, whatever the province.

Our health-care system also provides a significant number of reasonably good jobs, especially for women. Before medicare, hospitals and doctors could not count on payment from patients. Many hospitals and doctors alike functioned on the basis of charity, and they too often expected their workers to do the same. Now they have secure funding from governments and no pressure to show profits. Brought together in large organizations as funds flowed to hospital services, health-care providers have formed unions to help protect their rights and ensure that the quality of their working conditions allows them to provide good care. Meanwhile doctors enjoy guaranteed employment and payment, something that virtually no other occupation has.

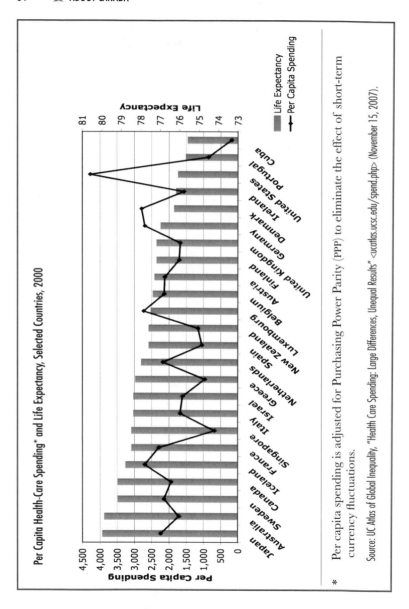

Per Capita Health-Care Spending* and Life Expectancy, Selected Countries, 2000

Life Expectancy

Per Capita Spending

* Per capita spending is adjusted for Purchasing Power Parity (PPP) to eliminate the effect of short-term currency fluctuations.

Source: UC Atlas of Global Inequality, "Health Care Spending: Large Differences, Unequal Results" <ucatlas.ucsc.edu/spend.php> (November 15, 2007).

Our universal health insurance program helps to control costs. The divergence in U.S. and Canadian costs started when we introduced our universal plan. Before then, at just over 7 percent of Gross Domestic Product (total economic output, or GDP), Canada's expenditures on care were quite similar to those south of the border. After the introduction of medicare in 1971, the growth in health-care costs in Canada has been modest while those in the United States have soared.[2] The Canadian figure is now about 10 percent, while the U.S. figure is well above 15 percent, and of course the U.S. system leaves many without care and produces no better health outcomes overall. A universal plan is by all measures more efficient not only because we dramatically reduce administrative costs but also because we can co-ordinate care across regions and services. Although we still have a long way to go to achieve fully integrated care, in part because there is so much private practice and ownership, our system is much more integrated than is the U.S. system.

Our universal system works to give us a competitive edge in international trade. Corporations in Canada save a great deal of money because they do not have to pay for most of their workers' health care now or in the workers' retirement. It is much cheaper to produce cars here, for example, than in the United States, and health-care costs are a decisive factor in this advantage. Indeed, health-care expenses constitute a major reason as to why GM in particular is in financial trouble. Similarly, individual bankruptcy as a result of prohibitive health-care debts is virtually unknown in Canada, while such debts are the most common cause of personal bankruptcy in the United States.

Neither Perfect Nor Perfectly Equitable

Medicare is not a perfect system, nor has it ever been a perfectly equitable one. It was designed in a time when doctors and hospitals were for most people the unquestioned centre of care. The *Canada Health Act* reinforced the focus on treatment and cure over prevention and health promotion by funding these services rather than others. People with psychiatric problems, for example, were frequently hospitalized instead of being treated in smaller facilities or at home. There was nothing to stop provinces from investing in other areas, although they could not count on federal funding to support such programs.

Although doctors and hospitals had little or nothing to stop them from promoting health and disease prevention, they had little incentive to do so either. Indeed, given that doctors were still paid on the basis of fee-for-service, they had an incentive to increase the emphasis on complicated, frequent treatment done as quickly as possible. In fee-for-service payment methods, each piece is paid a specific price—which means the more episodes, the more revenue. Equally important, more complicated intervention receives greater compensations. A Caesarean birth, for example, comes with a higher fee than does a vaginal birth. The fee-for-service system also does little to promote group practice, given that each doctor is treated as an independent recipient of income.

Nor has there been much incentive to encourage interdisciplinary teams in which doctors share the work with other health providers, such as nurses. In a hospital, for example, nurses are most often salaried employees whose pay comes out of the global hospital budget, but they work beside doctors who are paid a fee directly by the government for each procedure performed. Here, too, both provincial/territorial funders and physicians have been free to support interdisciplinary teamwork, but the *Canada Health Act* offered no incentive for them to do so.

In short, doctors have been left quite independent as well as quite powerful. They determine what is medically necessary and thus powerfully influence how hospitals operate. Doctors are free to determine where they set up their private practices, with guaranteed payment from their provincial/territorial plan, but with very little oversight of their expenditures. Not surprisingly, given that they have had to attend university in a large urban centre where they then make their social and professional contacts, few have chosen to locate in rural and Northern areas. The result has too often been underserviced communities. This underservicing by doctors has been made worse by the closure of community hospitals throughout the country. Most doctors are reluctant to locate in areas without the support that hospitals provide for them.

Another big gap in the *Canada Health Act* is its failure to address the issue of doctors, other health professionals, and health-care facilities operating outside medicare. The act's focus on hospitals and doctors also means that provinces and territories do not have to conform to its criteria when they develop other kinds of services or use other kinds of providers. When a patient leaves the hospital, but still needs care, the government will find it easier to charge fees or even to avoid paying for that needed care altogether. Provinces and territories can also avoid the criteria by redefining hospitals as those sites that provide only the most acute care, leaving other health-care facilities such as rehab centres beyond the protections afforded by the act. They can avoid the criteria when it comes to providers such as midwives and nurse practitioners. That's one reason why there are so few such providers in their public systems.

In addition, the *Canada Health Act* says nothing about the ownership of health-care organizations. When the legislation was introduced, virtually all hospitals in Canada were non-profit organizations. Most were run by religious or community groups, with some municipal, provincial, or federally owned institutions as well. What the legislation did was offer to support payment to hospitals, without specifying what kind of hospital. It can be argued that the spirit of the legislation requires non-profit care, and that such care was assumed when the legislation was introduced. The act does not provide explicit protection, however, against people making a profit out of government funds allocated for care. This silence has become increasingly important as health-care services have become highly profitable businesses, especially in the United States. These businesses are seeking areas for expansion and are supported in this search by free-trade regulations as well as by some current politicians and investors.

Similarly, the act says nothing about private insurance coverage. All provinces and territories allow private coverage of areas not included in their public plans, leaving plenty of space for profit. Five provinces go further, prohibiting the sale of private insurance for areas covered by public care. The logic of this prohibition is simple. If people pay extra, they will expect special treatment and access to care. They will expect to go to the front of the line based on money rather than on need. Because there are only a limited number of health-care providers, this means that everyone else moves back farther in the line. Moreover, the sale of private insurance to cover public care makes sense only if you also encourage more private care to respond to the needs of those who are paying directly.

Contrary to what one might expect, then, adding private, for-profit facilities alongside the existing non-profit ones lengthens rather than shortens average wait times for non-emergency procedures such as hip and knee replacement and eye laser surgery. If private payment accompanies the private delivery of care, the effect is simply to shift who gets care most quickly to those with the deepest pockets. The rest of us, as a consequence, wait longer.

Even if public payment is maintained, private, for-profit facilities will inevitably seek out and contract with the public authority for the easiest cases, in the process making the public delivery system appear to be less efficient. The private facilities may also try to sell medically unnecessary procedures along with the medically necessary ones, thus reducing the time available from the finite supply of surgeons and other health professionals to do what's needed. Doctors working in both sectors may have incentives to encourage their wealthier patients to go private by maintaining long waiting times in the public system. Although doctors need significant powers in order to use their medical knowledge appropriately, the system also needs to balance these powers in terms of the health-care interests of society as a whole.

Equally important, while the *Canada Health Act* sets out the conditions for federal funding, it does not guarantee stable funding of any sort. This silence has become obvious as successive federal governments have unilaterally introduced new funding formulas that cut back their contributions to the provinces. The 2002 Romanow Commission on the Future of Health Care made stable funding a central recommendation, on the grounds that provinces and territories could neither plan for nor reform the system without some guarantee that the money would be there. Moreover, without stable funding the federal government has little means of enforcing the act. Indeed, it has done little enforcement in recent years. Although in its 2004 agreement with the provinces and territories the federal government did commit to ten years of stable and enhanced cash transfers, in line with Romanow's recommendation, and notwithstanding that it once again provides significant and measurable financial support for medicare, the federal government continues to show little inclination to enforce the provisions of the act.

In addition, the *Canada Health Act* declares that there are to be no financial and other barriers to medically necessary care covered under its provisions. The array of other barriers is vast, and difficult if not impossible to eliminate entirely. For health care to be effective, we as whole persons, and not just our specific body parts, need to be taken into account. We are diverse along class, gender, cultural, linguistic, religious, sexual orientation, and other lines. Some facilities and education programs now offer training to providers to help them deal appropriately with this diversity. A 1997 Supreme Court decision ordered facilities to accommodate patients with hearing disabilities.[3] Some facilities have hired interpreters who assist Aboriginal Canadians and non-Aboriginal health-care providers to better understand each other, not only literally but also culturally.

Given that women make up the majority of patients and of those who take others to receive care, as well as the vast majority of providers, and given that women have long suffered from discrimination in health care, programs that are sensitive to their needs are essential. Some such programs are in place, but we still have a long way to go in reducing and removing the barriers in access to quality care presented not only by gender but also by place of origin, age, disability, sexual orientation, and racialization.

Another barrier that continues, and may have even increased with the most recent rounds of reform, is the geographical distribution of facilities and services. Hospitals have been closed, especially in rural areas of the country. The number of employed nurses declined between 1995 and 2004, and doctors continue to determine where they will locate. As a result, especially in the sparsely populated regions of this huge land, too many people find it difficult to get to care. Added to this difficulty is the question of waiting for services (see chapter 5).

The Symbol and the Critics

As a symbol, the *Canada Health Act* represents a commitment to collective care, to access to treatment—and equitable treatment at that—based on need rather than on ability to pay, and to choices for both patients and providers. It has been relatively successful in providing reasonable access to good-quality care. This success contributes to the popular support that has proven to be its best protection. It has also allowed provinces and territories to shape their own health systems while at the same time creating relatively uniform quality and access to hospital and doctor care.

When some of these jurisdictions call for the elimination or transformation of the act, then, as Alberta and Quebec in particular have on occasion done, it is not because it restricts them in terms of the design and structure of the system. It can only be because they reject one or more of the five principles, namely, universality, accessibility, comprehensiveness, portability, and public administration. It is important, then, always to demand to know which principle or principles the provincial and other critics seek to eliminate or weaken, and why.

Whether out of conviction or because they can read the public opinion polls, however, most politicians embrace the act. The problems arise when they are tempted to chip away at the application of its principles. They may, for instance, tighten the definition of what public hospitals are mandated to do, with the effect that patients are sent home quicker and sicker, where they usually have to pay for some or all of their medications and their home-care, rehabilitation, and medication costs.

While it may be appropriate to send some patients home from hospital earlier than was traditionally the case, the extra costs that these patients (or their private health insurers) must pay offend the act's principle of accessibility and point to its limitation in terms of comprehensiveness. This limitation is more clearly demonstrated by critical silences in the act that not only leave some people without appropriate care but also undermine our public health system. What we did not get from the legislation has in recent years become critically important.

Canada's focus on U.S. comparisons is understandable, given our familiarity with what almost all of us reject as an unfair and expensive system. But we could learn much from comparisons with various European systems, which cover broader ranges of services. Greater familiarity with European systems would also help us counter the specious claims by Canadian privatizers that the existence of various public-private mixes in Europe demonstrates that more private financing and delivery of care here would pose no threat to what we have in the public sphere. Almost all European countries cover more of the total health-care bill from the public purse than we do, in part because of their broader and more tightly regulated ranges of services. Many of them also provide more generous ranges of social services in general. The existence of higher levels of income support, and more affordable child care and public-transit services, for example, reduces the burden of small user fees for doctor visits.

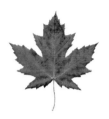

4. WHAT WE DID NOT GET

What we did not get in the *Canada Health Act* was the full range of services that Emmett Hall and other more recent commissions recommended. Yes, covering a wider range of services—home care and drugs, long-term residential care and various therapies, dentists, and alternative medicine—would require a significant initial investment on the part of governments. It would also challenge some vested interests. When medicare was introduced, the failure to cover these other aspects of care left room for for-profit insurance companies to offer benefits and opened up the space for other practitioners to set up practice. These companies and practitioners can charge whatever fees they want. While these groups and the people supporting market forces in all aspects of life resist extending the public system to these services, there are even more important reasons to do so now than there were in Hall's time.

Why Extend Medicare?

One important, continuing reason for covering the full range of services is equity. The *Canada Health Act* begins by stating that the main objective of health policy is to "protect, promote and restore the physical and mental well-being of residents of Canada and to facilitate reasonable access to health services without financial or other barriers." There is no logical reason, given this commitment, to limit this policy to hospitals, doctors, and a few other practitioners. Of course, a public system should be limited to necessary care, and this limitation will require decisions about what constitutes such necessary care. We cannot cover everything, but there can be little doubt that most long-term care and most drug expenditures, for example, are necessary. Yet, as soon as you leave the doctor's office or go out the hospital door, money more than need begins to influence who gets the services or the care. Once money becomes a factor, inequality is inevitable. If money should not be a barrier in access to doctors and hospitals, why should it be when it comes to home care, for example?

Another equally significant reason for including the full range of medically necessary services is to encourage the integration of the health system. If some parts of the system are in and some parts are out people will find it more difficult to move from one service to another. Overall planning becomes much more difficult to do, for both the patients and the providers. If the health-care system is to be fully effective and efficient from the patient's perspective, its vital components need to be integrated. The *Canada Health Act* promoted similar levels of doctor and hospital care across the country, creating the notion of medicare. When it comes to services outside the act, however, a great deal of variation exists across the country, creating in turn variations in accessibility.

Yet another reason is cost and efficiency. If the entire range of necessary services is to be part of the public system, the main reason for allocating people to one level of service becomes their health-care needs rather than who pays. Under the *Canada Health Act*, poor patients in a province that does not cover home care, for instance, may be kept in the more expensive hospital simply because they cannot pay for alternative care.

In addition, the payment system is necessarily more complicated when pieces are missing from care. The efficiencies that come with the single-payer system for doctors and hospitals are well documented.

They become particularly obvious when we compare Canada with the United States. Canada pays a third of what the United States pays on the cost of administering care. If medicare covered the full range of services, we could gain even more administrative efficiencies because the overhead costs of Canada's private health insurers are actually higher than those of private health insurers south of the border.[1] Equally important, if medicare covered the full range of services it could also save money by preventing illness or further deterioration. If people who have had knee surgery fail afterwards to get the required physiotherapy because they cannot afford the care, the surgery will probably also fail to have its proper effect, leading to the need for more care—and in the end bringing more suffering.

Missing as well is democratic decision-making and accountability.

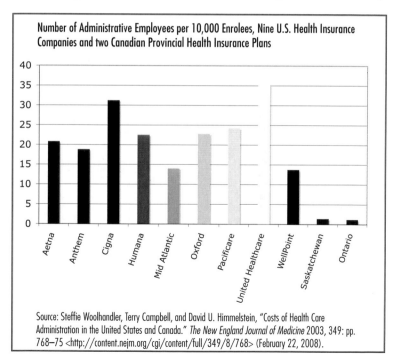

Number of Administrative Employees per 10,000 Enrolees, Nine U.S. Health Insurance Companies and two Canadian Provincial Health Insurance Plans

Source: Steffie Woolhandler, Terry Campbell, and David U. Himmelstein, "Costs of Health Care Administration in the United States and Canada." *The New England Journal of Medicine* 2003, 349: pp. 768–75 <http://content.nejm.org/cgi/content/full/349/8/768> (February 22, 2008).

A major benefit of a public system is the capacity to influence change through both elections and regular participation in community boards. Another is the ability to demand information on services and expenditures, along with a say in what those services and expenditures are. The system can be a collective and public process, rather than an individual one based on money and ability to pay. With some parts in and some critical parts out of the public system, Canadians find it difficult to participate in and to make assessments about care. With private insurers and providers come trade or commercial secrets, making accountability for the allocation of public funds that much more difficult if not impossible to achieve. It is also particularly difficult for those on low incomes to have choices about care.

Reforms undertaken over the last decade have made these missing pieces even more critical. Technological advances such as less invasive surgical procedures and new drugs have made it possible to dramatically reduce patient time in hospital, so that people are sent home quicker and sicker. Hospitals have had incentives in that regard, because government cutbacks reduce their income relative to the demands on them. Because the criteria of the *Canada Health Act* do not clearly apply when patients leave the hospital, governments can avoid the prohibition against user charges and extra-billing by moving people away from doctor and hospital care. At the same time, the kind of care that people need is changing. More people are surviving with disabilities; more are living well into old age. More workplace injuries create stress and strain, rather than broken bones and death, especially in female-dominated occupations. More politicians and corporate leaders promote less government and more market. It is therefore worth looking more specifically, at least briefly, at the missing pieces. Home care, pharmacare, and long-term care have received the most attention in recent years, but dental and eye care, midwifery, and alternative and complementary therapies are also among the missing.

Home Care

Home care is a popular topic of discussion in the media, and in many homes, as more and more care is shifted into the domestic sphere. Despite this widespread public discussion, as the Romanow Commission found, there is no one definition of home care, nor is there any consistency in what provinces and territories provide in terms of home-care services. Generally, the term is used to include one or more of three kinds of care: the paid services of visiting nurses and therapists; the provision of personal support care such as bathing and toileting; and other essential homemaking services such as cooking and cleaning, laundry, and meals. The purpose of home care may be to help people stay at home, rather than in a health-care facility. Or it may be to provide services that would otherwise be provided in long-term residential or institutional care. Increasingly the purpose is to support those who have been sent home quicker and sicker from hospital, including the growing numbers who have had day surgery.

The overwhelming majority of personal support and homemaking care is provided by people working without pay and most of these people are women. Many women want to provide this care, and many of those needing this care want to stay at home to get it. Increasingly, however, both patients and providers have less choice in the matter, as home care becomes the government's preferred option for where the care is to be provided, if not as a priority for public funding. In the words of the National Forum on Health, Canadian women react strongly against being "conscripted" into providing unpaid home care.[2] Increasingly, for both individuals and their care providers, financial resources determine both what choices they have and whether they get or give care. As a result, inequality grows. Genuine choice is available only to those with the ability to pay for alternatives.

Here the provinces and territories break all the principles set out in the *Canada Health Act.* All jurisdictions provide some assessment and some care management through the public system. All of them allow financial and other barriers to limit access to services. Some base home-care support on means tests to determine economic need, in the process denying universal access to this care. All permit fees for some supplies, drugs, and equipment. They thus fail to make home care comprehensive or reasonably accessible, and they fail to offer it under uniform terms and conditions. At least one province, Alberta, requires people to live within its borders for a year before becoming eligible for home care, rather than the three months set out in the *Canada Health Act* for doctor and hospital services. All of them require those seeking care to have a suitable home—a requirement that leaves out not only the homeless but also those living in rooming houses and some other living arrangements as well. The provinces and territories also have various ways of administering and delivering the programs, some of which make public scrutiny as required by the *Canada Health Act* difficult. This is the case in Ontario, with the bidding process that determines who delivers care. The Ontario government argues that the contracts signed by its local centres with the agencies providing home care must be kept secret to protect the competitive process.

Significant variations also exist across the country in who provides and who pays for care. In Manitoba home-care workers are public employees, but in most provinces home-care workers are employed by private organizations, some of them for-profit. Some provinces have virtually no cost-free home care. Some provinces will pay for homemaking services, while others will not. Some provinces charge fees for services that others provide without requiring any individual payment. Some provinces offer nursing care as long as patients need it, while others put time limits on this care. You could move across a provincial border and find that you are no longer able to get access to what was available in your home province. As a result of these variations, access to and quality of home care across Canada show significant inequities, just as doctor and hospital services did before medicare. Without shared principles of the sort provided in the *Canada Health Act*, the country has no universal access to home care.

Even though the *Canada Health Act* does not clearly identify home care as part of public care, governments cover the cost of most paid home care. According to estimates made for the Romanow Commission, governments pay about three-quarters of home-care costs. This estimate does not include the relatively insignificant amounts of home care covered by private insurance, which would somewhat reduce governments' share. Nevertheless, provincial governments are clearly already investing in home-care spending. On average, 5 percent of their health-care budgets go to home care, and these budgets are growing. Home care is clearly not the main priority, but it is still a significant amount of money—and we want our governments to spend that money wisely and equitably. Given that Canadians have a financial stake in home care, in addition to a vested interest resulting from our shared risk of needing or providing such care, we need to know how these dollars are spent.

Part of this investment goes to the administrative costs of applying means tests. Part goes to evaluating patients for eligibility, maximum hours, and other detailed criteria to determine who can get how much care, for how long, from whom. Denying care costs money—money that goes to administration rather than to care. Most provinces also spend money to co-ordinate care among the many providers. In addition, they spend money to determine who those providers are, because service is provided on the basis of limited contracts. In short, without a universal plan but with fees, the services cost more than they would if they were provided by government following the criteria found in the *Canada Health Act*. The system is not only more fragmented, but also more inequitable.

The money spent on home care increasingly goes to provide services for those leaving hospitals quicker and sicker or for those who would otherwise get treatment in hospitals. The techniques and drugs that allow people to be cared for at home do not end the need for highly skilled care. With limited budgets, home-care services give priority to those with the need for complex medical care. As a result, many of the disabled, those with chronic illnesses, and the frail elderly get less care, and less care than they need. This means that governments are also giving priority to treatment rather than to prevention. Homemaking services are usually the first to go. Yet good meals, as well as clean bathrooms and laundry, are critical factors in maintaining health and in preventing disease. In the long run, governments may well spend more on treating those made ill by their limitations. Different priorities in different regions in British Columbia allowed researcher Marcus Hollander to compare jurisdictions that cut back in homemaking with those that cut back on nursing. He showed that homemaking services were more important than nursing services in keeping care at home.[3] Of course, the reduction or elimination of this care also carries high costs for the individual in terms of personal dignity and health.

In short, our fragile and variable publicly paid-for home-care services perpetuate and even create inequalities among jurisdictions and individuals. Many of the most vulnerable people in our society are left without essential services while the priority is placed on those once provided for in hospitals. At the same time, the number of people needing home care is growing significantly in the wake of health-care reforms and changes in the patterns of both illness and age. Without a public system, the money we are investing is too often wasted on sorting the eligible from the ineligible while leaving too many without care.

The Romanow Commission recommended a national, public home-care plan based on the principles of the *Canada Health Act*. Begin, the Commission said, with limited mental health and after-hospital care, and care for the dying. This would establish a floor for services that provinces and territories would be free to build on. Undoubtedly, these additions would provide a more equitable system than what we have now. The problem is that this limited strategy is the same one that got us in trouble before. What was to be the first step in a full-service public health-care system was stalled at step two. As Hall made clear, providing the full range of services would be more equitable; it would also be more efficient because people will be provided with the most effective level of care.

Privileging those needing home care after they leave hospitals over those with the same needs resulting from chronic conditions certainly saves public funds in an immediate sense, because hospital care is so expensive. But it also offends the spirit of the *Canada Health Act*, because it allocates resources on the basis of cost considerations rather than on the basis of need. It probably also costs more in the long term, because those not receiving appropriate levels of home care are forced into long-term residential and hospital care sooner rather than later.

Pharmacare

As everyone who watches the commercials on U.S. television stations knows, prescription drugs, and not just over-the-counter medications, have become increasingly important and marketed components in health care over the last three decades. Drugs have allowed people to survive longer, to live more comfortably, to resist diseases, and to go home earlier from hospital or avoid hospital altogether. They have also become increasingly expensive. With more, and more expensive, drugs becoming central to care, a central issue becomes who pays.

The first Hall Commission on health care recommended that prescriptions drugs be included in public care. So have several investigations since then. We are still waiting. Although when we are in a hospital all of the drugs required for treatment are provided without cost to us as patients, we have no such guarantee once we leave the hospital. Outside hospitals, drug coverage in Canada looks much like health care in general does in the United States. Those on welfare have some drugs covered by the province or territory. So too do the elderly, the severely disabled, registered First Nations, some Inuit, and the military. The different provincial jurisdictions in Canada vary enormously in terms of coverage, payment and conditions. In 2003, for example, Newfoundland seniors poor enough to be eligible for the federal government's Guaranteed Income Supplement to their old age pensions did not pay for anything except the professional fee charged by pharmacists. But no other seniors in the province were covered. By contrast, in Alberta all seniors are covered under the provincial pharmacare plan, but they must pay 30 percent of prescription costs up to a maximum of $25 per prescription. Meanwhile, in Saskatchewan, all seniors are covered, and they all pay an annual contribution based on household income. According to the Organization for Economic Cooperation and Development, the only industrialized country with a lower public share of its prescription drug spending is the United States. At 68 percent in 2004 Germany, for example, placed fourth in this OECD ranking of twenty countries, covering from the public purse about double the share that Canada did. In eighth place, France was close behind Germany. Luxembourg, the Czech Republic, and Austria topped the rankings, in that order.[4]

Together, government drug plans account for about 46 percent of total prescription drug costs in Canada. Private insurance plans, usually acquired as part of an employment package, account for just over a third of costs—which still leaves individuals paying directly almost one-fifth of all drug expenditures. Some of this private expenditure results from the co-payments and deductibles on drug plans; some from no insurance coverage at all. The big, rich provinces tend not only to have more generous plans but also to have better employer coverage. People in the small Atlantic provinces are the most likely to pay for their own drugs.

As the Romanow Commission pointed out, the result is not only considerable variation across Canada but also considerable inequity. Where you live, where you work, and how old or how poor you are all influence access. Researcher Joel Lexchin found that these characteristics are in turn related to gender, racialization, class, and regions in Canada. Low-income people, for example, spend seven times as much of their incomes on pharmaceuticals as do high-income people.[5] The absence of a pharmacare program is particularly problematic for women given that they are prescribed more medications than men and are less likely than men to have drug coverage through paid work. With drugs prices escalating along with need, here is one health-care factor that could send a Canadian into personal bankruptcy. Tax-financed drug plans in British Columbia, Ontario, Manitoba, and Saskatchewan provide the best protection against very high drug costs. Yet many people even in those provinces may suffer financial hardship in order to get their required prescriptions. As is the case in the United States with medical care, many people simply go without. Even a five-dollar charge may be well beyond the means of a lone-parent woman living on welfare or an immigrant man earning a minimum wage in Toronto. Research in Quebec shows that when the province introduced co-payment fees for the poor and the elderly, essential drug use dropped and hospitalizations and physician and emergency room visits rose.[6]

Who pays is not the only question. What drugs are covered is also a critical issue in access and costs. Health Canada determines which drugs are safe for sale in this country, but the provinces and the territories have their own drug approval processes. Each establishes what is known as a formulary: a list of all drugs covered by its pharmacare program. The result is significant variation across the country in terms of which drugs are included as part of the tax-funded system. A person with Alzheimer's disease may have one drug covered in Ontario and a different one in British Columbia. The drug companies apply considerable pressure on the provinces to add their products to the formulary and to add them quickly. Especially when spurred by media reports of new miracle drugs, patients also pressure their provincial governments to pay for the particular drugs that they perceive they need. This pressure contributes to the variability.

There are good reasons to speed up the process of bringing new drugs to market. They may provide better care and a chance for recovery, avoid surgery, or ease pain for those without alternatives. Both pharmaceutical companies and some patients regularly appear in the media urging reforms that would bring new drugs more quickly to market and to the drug formularies. Health Canada has responded to these concerns by setting up a fast-track system for drugs that have the potential to save lives or address critical disabilities. Consequently, we are not denied access to drugs that can make a big difference by a lengthy approval process.

But there are also good reasons to take our time and make sure that drugs do what their promoters claim they do and do not create other risks. There are also good reasons to carefully evaluate which drugs are listed in formularies. Indeed, critical questions are already arising about the methods of approval in terms of their capacity to assess either benefits and risks or relative value. The assessment relies heavily on evidence produced by the company seeking to sell its drug. Its interests, which are mainly in profits, may conflict with those of patients and governments. Indeed, research has demonstrated this tendency in more than one case. There is now no easy way to hold Health Canada accountable to the public rather than to the drug companies, no easy way for the public to participate in decision-making or to appeal decisions.[7] That is why several investigations of the approval process have recommended the establishment of a body independent of both the government and the drug industry. As part of their 2004 federal/provincial/territorial accord on health, the first ministers agreed that we need an independent agency to evaluate the effectiveness and safety of new drugs for inclusion in the formularies. The country is still waiting for this recommendation to be put into practice.

Equally important are the criteria for assessing drugs. Drug companies do not have to demonstrate that their new products are better in either outcome or costs than are existing products. They simply have to demonstrate that they are better than nothing. The majority of drugs that appear on the market are often called line extensions: small variations on existing medications that allow the makers to take out a new patent that will prevent others from copying the drug, permitting the patent holder to charge more. Very few of the drugs introduced as new are new in any significant way other than price. Nor do drug companies have to follow the impact of a drug over time. While we cannot predict long-term side effects and risks with any accuracy, we can follow patients who are prescribed the drugs and monitor the results. For example, research shows that the arthritis drug Vioxx creates a relatively high risk of heart attacks. The risk became evident after approval, not during the examination of the drug for approval. After considerable debate, and after many deaths were attributed to the drug, Vioxx was finally withdrawn from the market.

The questions of which drugs are available on the market and which ones are on the drug formularies are in turn linked to price. Drugs prices are rising dramatically, along with a growth in the number of drugs sold. In all but two years since 1985, outpatient drug expenditures have risen significantly faster than the inflation

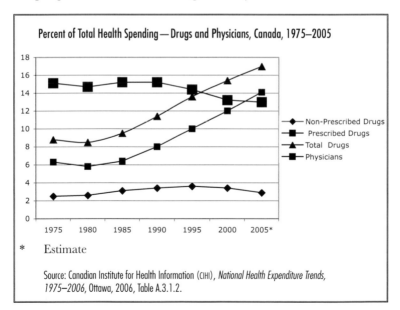

Percent of Total Health Spending — Drugs and Physicians, Canada, 1975–2005

—♦— Non-Prescribed Drugs
—■— Prescribed Drugs
—▲— Total Drugs
—■— Physicians

* Estimate

Source: Canadian Institute for Health Information (CIHI), *National Health Expenditure Trends, 1975–2006*, Ottawa, 2006, Table A.3.1.2.

rate.[8] Remember, governments already pay the largest share of drug costs. The price they pay, then, is critical to us all, even if we do not personally need the drug. The research-based drug companies, also known as the brand-name firms, argue that the high prices reflect the investments they make in creating life-saving drugs. Not only does such research cost a lot, but it is also risky because drugs that can consume years of expenses may fail to treat the problem, or they may carry too many other risks.

While it is appropriate that the drug companies seek a return on their investment, they are routinely the most profitable companies in the world. In 2002 the top ten drug companies on the Fortune 500 list of the world's largest companies had more combined net profits than did the other 490 companies.[9] The monopoly power they enjoy by being granted long-term patents for their products contributes greatly to their profitability. Meanwhile, the prices of patent drugs in Canada, while generally lower than those in the United States, are often much higher than prices for the same drugs sold in Europe, even though the same research costs apply everywhere.

In any case, much of the money that goes to basic research of the sort that leads to breakthroughs comes from governments, while the brand-name companies spend a great deal on drugs that simply create slight variations on old medicine. Sometimes called "evergreening," because it allows companies to retain the monopolies over the production and sale of their drugs long after the twenty-year patent has expired, this strategy is about profits rather than health. Not only that, but much of what the brand-name pharmaceutical companies claim as research expenditure is actually going to advertising and distributing the drugs. Marcia Angell, a doctor who teaches at Harvard Medical School and is a former editor of the *New England Journal of Medicine*, uses figures from the drug companies themselves to show that they spend less than 15 percent of their budgets on research, and over twice that much on marketing.[10]

Generic companies are another player in this field. They are the businesses that produce copies of drugs developed by others.

While the brand-name companies are large and foreign-owned, most generic firms are smaller, Canadian-based enterprises. This ownership matters, because the big international companies not only are more powerful but also often operate under different rules. Once Canada had drug prices second only to the United States. Following that old Canadian standby, a commission investigation, the government developed a process known as "compulsory licensing," which permitted the generic companies to copy drugs under a special permit while paying a royalty to those who developed it. As a result of the competition prices dropped to match those in Europe. Later investigation found that the research-based companies still made a handsome profit. Nevertheless, under pressure from those companies and from the negotiations for free trade with the United States, Canada eliminated the compulsory licensing system, extending the length of a patent and making the generic firms wait longer to copy a drug. Evergreening has the same effect. Meanwhile, it takes an average of eighteen to twenty months to get approval for a generic copy of a brand-name drug.

Total Health Expenditure by Use of Funds, Canada, 1975–2005 Percentages					
Year	Hospitals	Other Institutions	Physicians	Drugs (Prescribed)	All Other**
1975	44.7	9.2	15.2	8.8 (6.3)	22.2
1985	40.8	10.3	15.2	9.5 (6.4)	24.2
1995	34.4	9.7	14.4	13.6 (10.0)	27.9
2005*	30.1	9.4	13.0	17.0 (14.1)	30.5

*   Estimate.
** This category includes other health professionals (e.g., dentists), capital health spending, public health, health administration, and a miscellaneous category (e.g., home care).

Source: CIHI, *National Health Expenditure Trends, 1975–2006*, Ottawa, 2006, Table A3.1.2 — Part 2.

With compulsory licensing gone, the federal government did establish a Patented Medicine Prices Review Board (PMPRB), with the mandate of setting maximum prices for newly approved patented drugs. The maximum is the median list price for the drug in the United States, the United Kingdom, France, Germany, Italy, Sweden and Switzerland. This practice accounts for the generally lower prices in Canada as compared to the United States.

The share of total health spending devoted to drugs has grown dramatically. By 1997 it outstripped the share devoted to doctors, and by 2003 the share spent on prescription drugs alone exceeded that on doctors. Moreover, the drug spending share includes only the drugs taken outside hospital.

Not surprisingly, then, governments have been developing strategies to control drug costs. An increasingly popular strategy in government circles—but one proven to be ineffective in lowering costs to the public purse—is to introduce or increase co-payments and other user fees for those drugs covered by public programs. But some people cannot afford the extra charges, however low. By forgoing needed medications, they become sicker and end up needing more expensive care. Untreated diabetics, for example, are at serious risk of blindness, amputations, and heart attacks.

Another more effective strategy promotes the use of generic drugs over brand-name ones when they have the same impact. British Columbia pioneered this approach, called reference-based pricing, for selected, frequently prescribed drugs. What its provincial plan pays for is the lowest-price drug in a given therapeutic class. Patients can, but seldom do, top up the payment for a brand-name equivalent. This approach has saved the province millions of dollars while arousing a fierce backlash from the brand-name companies. The province has not extended the program beyond the five therapeutic classes introduced in its early years, and no other province has followed its initiative. More generally, the provinces have been reluctant to use their purchasing power to bargain aggressively for lower prices, even though they directly finance 42 percent of national prescription drug expenditures.[11]

Yet another strategy for reducing prescription drug costs involves cutting back on the demand for them. Canada restricts the direct-to-consumer advertising (DTCA) of prescription drugs. Such advertising stimulates inappropriate demand and inappropriate use. According to government policy, if a brand name such as Viagra is advertised, its intended use cannot be mentioned. This restriction is often infringed by the drug companies. You need only visit a woman's washroom to see advertising for birth-control pills.

Canadians also regularly see commercials on U.S. television and ads in U.S. magazines because the United States, alone in the world with New Zealand, has no such DTCA restriction. This border-crossing is used to justify the argument that the Canadian restriction should be dropped. CanWest MediaWorks, Canada's largest newspaper chain and the owner of the Global TV network, took the lead here by launching a lawsuit challenging the DTCA restriction on the grounds that it violates the protection of corporate rights to freedom of expression provided by the Charter of Rights and Freedoms.

On the other side are those who favour maintaining and even strengthening the DTCA restriction. Such advertising may contain exaggerated and misleading claims. It tends to downplay the potential harmful effects of the drug it promotes, and tends to discuss those effects in technical language that most lay consumers do not understand. It promotes particular brand names, and not the less expensive but equally effective older and often generic alternatives. It encourages people to start thinking that they have problems, or problems of greater severity, that can best be treated with drugs. Rather than inventing drugs to treat illness, on occasion the industry invents illnesses (or at least syndromes) to market drugs. Instead of a pill for every ill, there's an ill for every pill. A prominent DTCA example is "sexual dysfunction," to be treated with Viagra, Cialis, or a similar brand-name drug.

In response to public criticism, the brand-name drug industry introduced a voluntary policy aimed at limiting the lavish gifts and free trips that drug companies have traditionally offered to physicians. Those gifts and trips have, of course, been offered because they are effective in influencing the prescribing behaviour of physicians, sometimes in inappropriate ways and certainly in expensive ways. More generally, in response to the overprescribing that is all too common, especially for women and for seniors of both sexes, governments and professional organizations are undertaking initiatives to educate both physicians and patients. Electronic health records are being used to track prescribing patterns, and seniors in particular are being urged to bring to a nurse or doctor at regular intervals all the drugs they are taking. Pharmacists are also playing an increasingly critical role in advising both patients and prescribers about drugs and their interactions.

A final approach, which could be combined with all the others, is to develop a national pharmacare strategy modelled on the *Canada Health Act*. It has long been observed that without universally accessible coverage for medically necessary drugs, not only is medicare grievously incomplete but also drug spending is needlessly expensive for society as a whole. Without "first-dollar" coverage outside hospital at no cost to the user, some people are denied the health care they need. A national pharmacare program would be more equitable and cheaper than what we now have in place. It would reduce the costs associated with advertising, administration, profits, and drug-pricing that plague the mix of public and private approaches. It would allow bulk purchasing and promote shared formularies.

A national pharmacare program could, at the same time, encourage the more rational use of drugs and the more rational selection of those drugs to be used. As is the case now with doctor and hospital care, the public purse would cover the cost of necessary drugs with a demonstrated benefit. This does not mean that all drugs would be paid for. Some selection would still be required, but it would mean more equitable access to those drugs assessed to be useful.

There is bound to be controversy here. Patients with life-threatening conditions who are not responding positively to existing drugs have little to lose from demanding access to new drugs that have not (yet) been shown to be more effective than the existing ones. Costing as much as several thousand dollars a month, these drugs are typically much more expensive. Their inclusion in a pharma-care formulary would thus come at the expense of other kinds of spending, whether in health care or elsewhere, whether in the public sector or the private. Exclusion from a public formulary raises the further question of whether medicare (that is, hospitals and doctors) should be used for the administration of these drugs. Either patients who are prepared to pay for them are denied access, or the public system becomes explicitly complicit in the provision of care on the basis of ability to pay rather than need: a difficult choice. Cancer Care Ontario, a provincial government agency, proposed the second option, arguing that it is impractical as well as politically unpalatable to deny access to new drugs that some desperate patients want, even though those drugs might turn out to be ineffective.

Indeed, many drugs that are now available are not just of un-doubted benefit but also very costly. In uneven fashion, provinces and territories assume some or most of the costs for some or most of what are called "catastrophic" drugs, which are "medications so expen-sive or used in such quantities that they cause financial hardship."[12] Although disagreeing on the details, both the Romanow Commission and the Kirby Committee recommended step-by-step moves towards pharmacare, with a national catastrophic drug plan as the next step. The 2004 first ministers meeting, at which the federal government agreed to transfer an additional $41 billion to the provinces and territories, also saw agreement in principle on the establishment of a catastrophic plan. Researchers have estimated how far the various provinces would have to go to protect Canadians from catastrophic drug costs,[13] and governments insist that such an approach remains a high priority. But a plan has yet to be enacted.

Again, a plan might follow the same trajectory taken with hos-pital and then medicare care: beginning with one element and with the intention of moving on to include other necessary elements in later stages. The danger is that we will stop at the first stage, having partially addressed the most immediate threat to personal bankruptcy. Stopping there could also mean continuing inequity, even for catastrophic drug costs. Someone working full-time at the minimum wage in Ontario, for example, would be below the poverty line but still required to spend $425 a year on drugs before reaching the catastrophic threshold recommended by the Kirby Committee. To pay that much for drugs would mean giving up essentials such as food. Recognizing this issue, a 2006 report to the federal/provincial/territorial governments recommended a sliding scale of payments, further reducing but not eliminating what the poor would have to pay.[14]

After the 2004 meeting, the first ministers also began working on plans for the development of new and expensive drugs to treat rare diseases, a national formulary, pricing and joint purchasing strategies, and the "real world" evaluation of the safety and effectiveness of drugs after their approval by Health Canada. Progress on these plans has been slow, partly because of jurisdictional difficulties. Quebec is not part of the first ministers' efforts, and with much of the brand-name pharmaceutical industry located within its borders the provincial government there is particularly adamant that Ottawa stay out of its jurisdiction. Other provinces, especially the larger, richer ones, are also at times resistant to further federal involvement, although the premiers did propose in the summer of 2004 that jurisdiction and responsibility for pharmacare be taken over by the federal government. The federal government rejected the proposal.

Pressure from the powerful pharmaceutical companies and from the insurance companies that cover these costs also makes progress difficult. When Ontario tried to take small steps in this direction in 2006, it ran straight into this pressure. Despite evidence supporting its efforts, the province quickly backed off from most of its initial steps for controlling drug costs.

But this does not mean there is no hope for change. Corporations that provide health benefits to their employees are also facing rising costs, and they have learned from medicare that it is cheaper to share costs across the entire population. Equally important is the growing public support for such a plan as drugs prices rise. The Canadian Health Coalition, which brings together unions with community and faith organizations, is working hard to bring about the extension of medicare to drugs coverage, as Hall recommended, just as the organization did in the years leading up to the *Canada Health Act.*

A national pharmacare plan has been the subject of recommendations for years—and it has been backed by popular demand. A national pharmacare plan would improve access and equity. It would also help control the already large amounts that governments spend on drugs, especially if they use their considerable clout to reduce prices and rigorously assess drugs to be included in a single, national formulary. But powerful vested interests resist progressive reform and demand even greater freedom to raise and control prices.

Long-Term Care

Long-term care represents another big hole in the *Canada Health Act.* Facilities for people who need long-term care are nothing new in Canada. Ontario had them more than a century ago. Nor is the proportion of the population in such facilities now much different than it has ever been. What is new is the care required in these facilities. With hospitals keeping only the most acute cases, many of those once cared for in hospitals are now being sent to long-term care facilities. With home care being used to keep people at home as long as possible, long-term care facilities are no longer dominated by frail, elderly women. Instead, those now in long-term care facilities are mostly the very old who have complex medical and mental problems that require constant and considerable care. With fewer chronic care and psychiatric hospitals, more and more long-term care residents are young people with long-term, multiple medical issues who are too ill to be cared for at home.

As is the case with both home care and drugs, governments have made a considerable public investment in long-term care facilities. Thus, Canadians in general have an economic and social interest in who gets care, of what quality, and at what cost. The *Canada Health Act* defines hospitals as places that provide acute, rehabilitative, or chronic care, but not as providing nursing home intermediate care, adult or child residential care, or care for those defined as mentally ill. Sending people to long-term care facilities seems to provide a way in which governments can avoid the principles of the act, and they do. All provinces charge some fees for care, often for services explicitly covered in the act for hospital care. Equally important, the share paid by governments differs from jurisdiction to jurisdiction. In Ontario, for example, the public purse pays for nursing care but not for what is called accommodation and meals. There is also considerable variation across Canada in terms of eligibility for care. As a result, there is no universal coverage nor are there uniform terms and conditions. Care, then, is neither comprehensive nor accessible. With different rules from jurisdiction to jurisdiction, long-term care is also not portable from province to province.

Government payments are matters of record, although those records are often difficult to decipher. With private, for-profit organizations increasingly delivering long-term care, there is less openly public administration of the facilities. Even the contracts that involve the use of government funds may be secret. We do know that staffing levels in British Columbia's not-for-profit nursing homes, for example, are significantly higher than those in the province's for-profit homes. Research has shown that higher staffing levels result in better care outcomes, up to a threshold of 4.1 hours of care by nurses and care aides per resident per day.[15]

In the waves of reforms that altered who entered long-term care facilities, little was done to make these places better. Indeed, some initiatives made them worse. In Ontario, for example, the Conservative government of the 1990s removed the regulations that required a minimum of 2.25 hours of daily nursing care per resident and the requirement that at least one registered nurse be on duty at all times. Still, there are some signs of improvement. The Liberal Party won the 2006 election in New Brunswick with a pledge to move to a minimum of 3.5 hours. Saskatchewan has a minimum of 3.1 hours, and Nova Scotia is raising its minimum to 3.25 hours. Ontario did not include a minimum in Bill 140, its 2006 legislation on long-term care, but did include random surprise inspections, the recognition of family councils, protection for whistle-blowers, and some restrictions on the use of restraints.

If sixty has become the new fifty, long-term care facilities have become the new hospitals for many people. Yet these particular hospitals have been defined out of the *Canada Health Act* and provided under unequal conditions across Canada. The two richest provinces, Ontario and Alberta, have been chastised by their auditors general for failing to invest enough in such care and for failing to ensure quality care. Others have faced increasing public outrage at what is happening to people in these care facilities. A few whistle-blowers brave enough to expose conditions have made headlines, as have some cases taken on behalf of patients who have received inadequate, or even outrageous, care. These facilities often have such a poor reputation that few enter them by choice, and many families feel incredible guilt when their relatives do enter one. Instead of focusing on making them good places for public care, though, government and often community energies have focused on keeping people out of them.

> "Neglect of aged an 'outrage,'" blares the lead headline in *The Toronto Star* of October 4, 2007. "Provincial politicians challenged to relieve nursing home suffering or face legal action," reads the sub-headline. The reason? Government regulations require the homes to keep their residents "clean and dry" and to "promote their dignity and independence." Yet a common practice in these homes is to keep residents in wet diapers until the diapers are 75 percent full of urine.

Dentists and Eye Doctors

Although the *Canada Health Act* does explicitly name physician care, most dental and some eye care are not considered part of public health plans. This is particularly surprising today, given that health promotion is increasingly the talk of governments seeking to reform health care. The research by Dennis Raphael and others clearly demonstrates that health is influenced primarily by food, shelter, jobs, joy, and income, factors that taken together are usually called the determinants of health.[16] For instance, studies suggest that the distribution of income in a given society may be a more important determinant of health than the total amount of income earned by society members. Large gaps in income distribution lead to increases in social problems and poorer health among the population as a whole.[17] One group of researchers point out: "In the 1994 National Longitudinal Survey on Children and Youth (NLSCY), families headed by single-mothers were eight times more likely to report that their children were hungry, compared to other families. Children from families receiving welfare were 13 times more likely to experience hunger than non-welfare families."[18] Based on this research and seeking ways to save costs in the long run, multiple reports advise a shift from treatment to prevention and health promotion. Yet most of the emphasis has been on prevention as defined in medical terms. It is tests and treatment, rather than social programs such as income supports, that are the primary focus of concern in health circles.

Even with this narrow focus, however, two effective medical interventions are receiving even less government support. Justice Emmett Hall long ago recommended that dentists and eye exams be included as part of the medicare package. The *Canada Health Act* mentions dentists, but only within the context of hospital care. There is no universal coverage for either of these important prevention strategies. As with other health services, all jurisdictions provide some public services. Quebec, for example, once covered annual checkups and basic dental care for children. Ontario covered most eye examinations. Both provinces, along with Manitoba, have since delisted these services for most of the population, introducing much stricter guidelines about who can get care paid for from the public purse. Across the country, governments have been retreating from the limited coverage they once had.

Complementary and Alternative Medicines

Health care is dominated in Canada by allopathic medicine: a system focused on the penetration of the body physically by surgery and chemically by drugs. In allopathic medicine, the emphasis is on fixing a body part based on the assumptions that what is mainly a biologically determined problem can be addressed by experts trained on the basis of evidence understood as scientific. This approach is so dominant in Canadian health care that we have come to think of it as all of health care. Indeed, it is virtually the only kind of health care supported by the public health scheme.

But there are other ways of approaching health, illness, and disability. There are also other ways of understanding evidence. Chiropractic, homeopathy, acupuncture, and massage therapy are just four of what are often called complementary and alternative medicines. Each is developed from an evidence base different from the sort used in allopathy. Indeed, each is often criticized on the grounds that its approach is not based on evidence such as the double-blind randomized clinical trials that are seen as the gold standard in allopathic medicine. A double-blind, randomized clinical trial is one in which neither the patients nor the providers know if the patient is taking or undergoing the intervention being tested or whether they are having something else, like a sugar pill. Such research first of all requires an intervention of a particular sort, which is more typical of allopathic than of other forms of therapy. It also requires the assumption that you can influence one part of the body to determine cause and effect, without having an impact on other parts of the body. This is also an assumption not always found in other forms of care.

Complementary and alternative medicines often start from a different set of assumptions, ones that are frequently rejected by allopathic medicine. These different assumptions, combined with the threat of competition, have contributed to the strong opposition sometimes voiced by doctors towards these practitioners. Their opposition has been one factor in the failure to include them in medicare. Nevertheless, many Canadians find the alternative and complementary medicines useful, and some people even find them superior to the allopathic approach.

Despite the allopathic dominance, some complementary and alternative approaches are recognized in public plans. Ontario covers a limited number of chiropractic visits, for example, although this coverage too has been reduced in recent years. Insurance companies also include some coverage for approaches such as massage therapy. For the most part, however, Canadians cover complementary and alterative medicines out of their own pockets.

Although governments have prevented some alternative providers from offering their services in the name of safety, they have left other providers largely alone. Practitioners have enjoyed only limited success in seeking recognition as registered health professions. Such registration brings legitimacy, because it simultaneously acknowledges that the approach is indeed a useful health profession and ensures that those practising are duly qualified. In 2004 the federal government moved to regulate some of the alternative medicines. This move too serves to legitimate the medicine at the same time as it seeks to ensure safety.

For the most part, then, complementary and alternative medicines operate outside both public and private insurance plans. Some operate outside government regulation as well.

Contravening the Five Principles

What we did not get with the *Canada Health Act* was equity, although we did get significantly more equity than we had before medicare.

Location still matters in health services, with urban dwellers often receiving more, better, and faster care. Other social locations such as membership in racialized groups, gender, and disability also still matter, although here, too, we have made progress in terms of hospital and doctor care. Nor did we get a problem-free system or one that is always on top of the latest developments. We did, nevertheless, get the possibility of dealing with these problems collectively and democratically

More obviously, we did not get the full range of service recommended by Hall and by others. The public purse pays for a lot of drugs and long-term care, for some home care, dental work, and eye care, and for a few complementary approaches to care. But in each of these cases, the five principles of the *Canada Health Act* are contravened. Care is not universally available; it is not accessible without financial or other barriers; it is not comprehensive within each service; it is not portable; and it does not meet the criteria for public administration. The result is not just much greater inequality in access than is the case for doctors and hospitals. It is also higher administrative costs, less co-ordination, and more waste in terms of the appropriate allocation of care.

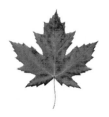

5. REFORMING PRIMARY CARE

Years ago the World Health Organization defined primary health care as the first level of contact of individuals, the family, and the community, bringing health care as close as possible to where people live and work. Primary care should provide promotive, preventive, curative, supportive, and rehabilitative services and constitutes the first element of a continuing health-care process.[1] This broad definition encompasses everything from a physician in solo practice to a community health centre where teams of providers are concerned with social development as well as individual health care, and are governed by an elected board. It suggests a common commitment to serving whole persons, close to their homes where everyone knows their names and circumstances. It suggests as well an emphasis on keeping people healthy and, when this fails, on providing a smooth and comforting transition to appropriate treatments. Although we did get public primary care with medicare, the form it took reflects a victory for many doctors and a reinforcement of physician-centred care rather than support for the kind of primary care indicated by the World Health Organization definition.

Problematic Primary Care

In Canada most people now come to the health-care system through their doctor's office. Most of these doctors work on a fee-for-service basis, often alone but now more frequently with other doctors in shared facilities. Since the earliest days of medicare, however, some people have received care through community health centres. Indeed, a few such centres existed before medicare and were supported because they offered advantages in both care and costs. Some of the problems with fee-for-service medicine, especially when combined with solo practices or group practices organized solely to share business services, were obvious when medicare was established. Other problems have emerged in more recent years.

For one thing, payment on the basis of each piece of service encourages physicians to provide as many services as they can, as quickly as they can. This can in turn lead to an undue reliance on prescription drugs, diagnostic tests, and other approaches designed to address specific symptoms in specific body parts. Moreover, more complex treatments tend to pay more, producing a perverse incentive to the provision of excessive interventions. This can lead to increased rates of hospital admission for expensive tests and procedures. The consequences may be both higher costs for the system and less appropriate care for the patient. By rewarding activity to address specific diagnoses and treatments and by failing to pay for more time on complex interactions, the fee-for-service system discourages physicians from spending time with their patients to explore multiple causes of ill health or to identify disease prevention and health promotion strategies. Equally important, it discourages primary care providers from holding team meetings to discuss patient issues.

This tendency is reinforced by medical education. Physicians are, in the main, trained to provide diagnosis and treatment to individuals, with an emphasis on specific body parts. They are oriented to medical intervention, medical preventive care, and medical means for maintaining good health. Yet the research on health promotion and disease prevention clearly demonstrates that good health is determined by multiple, interacting factors that need to be addressed in a variety of ways. Many of these social determinants of health involve skills well beyond medical care, and some require an understanding of

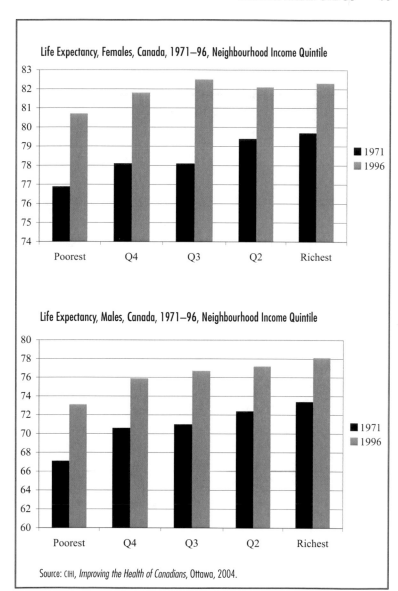

Life Expectancy, Females, Canada, 1971–96, Neighbourhood Income Quintile

Life Expectancy, Males, Canada, 1971–96, Neighbourhood Income Quintile

Source: CIHI, *Improving the Health of Canadians*, Ottawa, 2004.

the communities in which people live. The skills of physicians alone are inadequate to the task of promoting good health. The emphasis on solo medical practices fails to take advantage of the full range of provider skills, skills that are critical to both promoting health and treating illness or disability.

Many of these skills are difficult to see, mainly because they are often assumed to come naturally to the women who are the overwhelming majority of care providers. Moreover, no single physician can hope to maintain a command of the rapidly growing and increasingly available evidence on diagnosis and treatment, let alone the burgeoning research literature on the social determinants of health. Working alone, or in a group practice designed to share costs rather than care, can isolate such physicians and place too much responsibility in their hands.

Yet another problem presents itself with solo practice and fee-for-service payment. The system provides little opportunity for others to monitor physicians' work, to raise their concerns, or contribute their knowledge. Doctors in group practices are often organized primarily to promote business efficiency rather than shared knowledge and feedback. To invoke a currently fashionable term, there is little scope for "accountability." This is especially the case for physicians who lack hospital admitting privileges. With those privileges at least some other care providers see them at work and others are there to share information and offer advice.

Finally, it is difficult for even a small group of physicians, let alone a single physician, to cover more than a limited number of working hours each week. While illness and injury have never kept regular working hours, the demand for longer office hours has increased now that a majority of both women and men have paid work, that more of their paid work is precarious, and that more of it is undertaken on weekends and evenings. Moreover, especially with the increasing number of women working as physicians while retaining disproportionate domestic responsibilities, more and more physicians are seeking regular working hours and benefits. Then too, with patients leaving hospitals quicker and sicker and with a smaller proportion of the frail admitted to long-term care, the demands for services at all hours from doctors and clinics is growing. Moreover, solo and small-group practices cannot readily afford the kinds of equipment and facilities required to provide the full range of essential services set out in the World Health Organization definition of primary care. In particular, the rapidly developing information technologies offer new possibilities for searching the research literature, tracking patients, and communicating with other providers. But these technologies are expensive and thus are more accessible to larger organizations. The shift during the early part of the twentieth century to hospital-based care was in part a result of similar technological pressures.

Most recently, health-care restructuring has meant that more care is provided in the community in ways that increase the pressure on primary care services. There are greater discontinuities in services as patients are moved rapidly among institutions and across facilities. At the same time, emergency rooms are being redefined. Now only the most urgent, acute, and complex care is defined as being appropriately provided in these facilities. This new definition of hospitals and their emergency rooms is matched by increasing pressure on primary care providers to be open all hours. Meanwhile, new technologies make it possible for primary care organizations to seek advice from specialists or to obtain patient information rapidly and effectively through electronic means. It is thus easier to offer a wider range of services through primary care sites and easier to provide services to people at home, especially through twenty-four-hour, seven-day-a-week telephone advice systems that inform callers immediately on how they should address problems and on whether and where they should seek outside care or support.

For all these reasons and more, primary care has been the focus of investigations and of strategies for reform. Together, they offer an important opportunity to develop a health-care system that better responds to the needs and wishes of Canadians today. But they also create the possibility of a transformed system that is less accessible, more technocratic, and less responsive to what citizens need and want.

Promising Primary Care

The proposed and already implemented primary care reforms have many positive aspects. Specifically, there is now considerable pressure to eliminate the perverse incentives created by fee-for-service remuneration and the problems inherent in solo medical practice. The emphasis on interdisciplinary practice could serve to enhance the skills and accountability in practices while increasing access by sharing the physician's work.

Nurses, social workers, pharmacists, nursing aides, and others have much to offer in primary care. This is particularly the case if health promotion is defined to include more than medical interventions and self-care. The research on health promotion clearly demonstrates that a host of factors beyond the practice of medicine influence health. Health Canada, for instance, lists eleven additional factors, including social support networks, income and social status, healthy child development, employment and working conditions, and culture. These factors can best be addressed by recognizing and bringing together the complementary skills of many different providers. We cannot expect physicians alone to have the wide range of required skills. We can, however, create teams in which these skills are combined in ways that are designed to complement each other rather than create new hierarchies of care.

Equally important, the reform proposals emphasize health promotion and disease and injury prevention, along with at least a formal recognition of the social determinants of health. These proposals are combined with efforts to make care not only more continuous, especially through the use of new information technologies, but also available twenty-four hours, seven days a week. This approach, too, could expand access and reduce inappropriate use of emergency room services. Alternative payment systems, such as salaries for physicians, could support both team work and health promotion. Doctors and other team members would not have to think primarily in terms of money when they take time to promote health and to discuss care with teams. Current practices, such as fee-for-service payment going to doctors only, can severely limit this potential.

Risky Reforms

Although the WHO definition is often embraced in general terms, the central focus in practice is usually on the diagnosis and treatment of diseases and injuries by physicians.[2] In general, the Canadian strategies emphasize the need to organize family physicians and general practitioners into group practices. Current reform proposals remain largely centred on physicians, with group practices expanded to include, in subordinate positions, nurses and perhaps other providers. Nurse practitioners and possibly midwives, occupational therapists, and physiotherapists are to take over some of the physicians' tasks and to "provide patient education to support self-care," as physician Walter Rosser and nurse Jan Kasperski, the authors of one reform proposal, put it.[3] The focus would still be on the medical model, with its emphasis on the curative care of discrete body parts. There is little emphasis in the proposals on teamwork based on the complementary skills offered by different types of health providers. Instead, the model could well mean that nurses end up doing what doctors do not want to do, or what they are not available to do at night or in remote areas. Yet it is just such teamwork that has enabled community health centres to serve whole people in the contexts of their households and communities.

Alternative payment systems for physicians may also have a negative side. A central strategy is payment per patient rather than per intervention. Individual patients would be enrolled into group or individual practices. The funding of these practices would be based on the total number of patients enrolled and their characteristics, such as age and sex.[4] Each patient would have one entry point for services, and new information technologies would be introduced to track patients through the services they received and the costs they incurred. The idea is that continuity in care would be ensured by enrollment, with each enrolled patient served by the same practice over time.

Many current proposals would require patients to enroll with one physician-based practice, and they or their physician's practice would be penalized for their use of other primary care services. Rules for allowing limited exceptions would be established, but in general each of us would be restricted to just one "choice." Patient choice in most models means, as Rosser and Kasperski put it, that "every person would choose one family physician and that partnership would be formalized."[5] The opportunity to seek a second opinion, or to use different providers for different purposes, would be severely restricted.

Under our system now, Canadians have the right of access to any doctor or hospital, subject only to the limitations created by the numbers available and the requirement for a referral to a specialist, or to most diagnostic services, from their primary care physician. This choice results directly from our decision to fund services rather than individuals, and it has been a major source of the popular support for the Canadian public health system. It leaves us with more choices in terms of providers and services than either British or U.S. citizens get in their systems.

This is not to suggest that Canadians are now constantly "doctor shopping." The overwhelming majority—between 80 and 90 percent—can name their personal physician,[6] and thus now have continuity through their main care provider. In other words, the data suggest that for the most part patients already practise what the proposed restrictions are meant to achieve. By formalizing the practice, however, the reforms would make it more difficult to consult a different provider when there is good reason to do so. One good reason for seeking other services is that travelling for work, education, or holidays may take you far from your normal services. Another is the occasional need for a second opinion. A third is the legitimate desire to have a particular service provided by someone outside one's regular practice. For example, a young woman may not want to ask her family's clinic about birth control or have her tests for sexually transmitted diseases done there, but does want to stay with that practice for her other health needs. A fourth, but far from final reason, is the incapacity of the providers in a particular clinic to diagnose or treat a specific problem. Patients may be frustrated by its failure to treat a chronic complaint but happy with the rest of the health services in the practice. These choices made by individual patients can be more efficient and effective for the system as a whole in the long run. The appropriate reasons for seeking alternatives to one's regular services cannot be addressed by the right to change doctors with six months' notice, as some reform strategies suggest. If large numbers of patients are not now inappropriately moving around among services, why institute a reform that would so dramatically limit their choices?

At the same time, the enrolling or rostering of individuals would fundamentally transform access to health care. All residents of a province or territory now belong to its health plan and have the right of access to any service, either directly or on referral from their primary care physician. This condition not only allows residents choice, but also ensures that they will not be denied access because they have not enrolled with a particular practice or with its connected services. Indeed, many patients may find it difficult to enroll, and regularly to re-enroll, as the insured who enjoy "choice" must now do in the United States. Patients with severe or chronic diseases or injuries might be shunned by provider organizations, as might those whose language or culture is not that of the dominant majority. Marginalized populations such as the homeless and those with low literacy levels, and those with special needs, might be particularly at risk. Women may experience more difficulties gaining access, because they tend to use more health-care services than men do. Thus, a failure to enroll may not be the fault of a patient. It can result from the actions or inactions of provider organizations, especially if they have any incentives to deny or avoid the enrollment of individuals whose care could be expensive.

Equally important, rostering individuals opens up the possibility of denying individuals the care they might need, because the door at the single entry point may be closed. This could be the result of a misdiagnosis or of a shortage of spaces for new enrollees at the practices in a community. The group practice model now being promoted as the model, supplemented by clinics in rural areas and facilities closer to the existing nursing stations in remote areas, suggests a tiered model of primary health services. Multiple entry points in all areas where they are possible would better provide for a more flexible primary care system, without creating one kind of service for the rich, urban and well, and other systems (or none) for the poor, rural, and ill.

Moreover, rostering entails substantial administrative costs in recruiting and registering individuals, in transferring and recording when patients do change providers, and in sorting out the eligible from the ineligible. One reason why U.S. health care is so much more expensive is because it spends so much money tracking rostered patients and sorting the deserving from the undeserving. That necessity is linked to another problem. The rationale for rostering is to enable a shift from fee-for-service to per-head or capitation funding, which brings with it its own problems. The numbers of enrolled patients and their health-related characteristics would become the basis for group practice payment. With funding following individuals rather than services, the idea is that physicians would become more committed to providing continuous care that keeps their patients healthy. This would reduce diagnosis and treatment costs, thus increasing physician income and reducing their workloads.

Such is the theory. However, the problem with rostering evident in the United States is that the perverse incentive associated with fee-for-service medicine (too much care) is replaced by a perverse incentive that is worse (too little care). Capitation encourages providers to avoid care that is costly but often appropriate and to avoid patients perceived to be costly because they are in need of care. While regulations could be introduced to prevent primary care providers from refusing patients and denying them treatments, experience from the United States clearly shows that there are many ingenious ways of avoiding heavy-care patients. Indeed, this experience has given rise to new terms such as "cherry-picking" and "cream-skimming." For example, patients may be invited to enroll by attending a breakfast meeting held on the second floor of a building with no elevator, an approach that eliminates the mobility-impaired and the frail. Such creative means of avoiding the regulations have given rise to a new genre of novels and movies that decry the denial of needed care by Managed Care organizations. Their "risk management" techniques calculate the monetary cost to the corporation of denying care compared to the cost of providing it in particular cases. The firms thus determine whether it pays to provide the service or to pay damages to the few who, when they are denied, successfully pursue lawsuits.

Many of the group practices are like the Managed Care schemes that have aroused so much criticism in the United States. If Canadian providers are to be saddled with the risks of paying for patients in poor health, they may turn to those with experience in coping with such risks. The results could be not only more sophisticated managed denial, but also the entry into Canadian health-care delivery of for-profit U.S. firms. Capitation and rostering fit nicely with the U.S. approach, making Canadian group practices forced to engage in risk management ripe for takeover. We have little reason to feel secure that the tradition of Canadian medicare will protect us, because the provisions of NAFTA and other international "trade" agreements may make these U.S. corporations very difficult to resist or remove.

Nor is it clear that the primary care reforms now being initiated will make providers more responsive to patients and more responsible practitioners. Most proposals for primary care reform still define accountability primarily in terms of making physicians responsible to other physicians, and perhaps to some managers. Patients are to have a say only in selecting where they enroll, and without elected community boards little or no formal provision exists for their continuing input and assessment. Neither other providers nor communities feature prominently in the accountability discussions in the proposals. Quebec has, however, demonstrated that it is quite feasible to have elected boards representing patients, providers, and managers, complemented by special provision for particular populations served by its local health and social service centres (CLSCs). Most pilot projects on primary care reform contain no provision for broad accountability, and the most recent federal-provincial agreement pays little attention to public participation in the construction of the report cards that are intended to enhance accountability.

Most proposals place a new emphasis on what is called evidence-based decision-making. Although evidence can provide useful guidelines for what physicians and other providers should do, it can also lead to rigid rules that substitute for decision-making based on an understanding of individuals in their particular social contexts. The U.S. accounting firm Milliman and Robertson recommends that doctors meet predetermined and quantified quality targets. It offers the example of aspirin, suggesting that because we can determine that it is desirable for all those who have had a heart attack to take aspirin, doctors should be paid partly on the basis of meeting a quality target for documented aspirin orders for these patients.[7] While guidelines based on aspirin research can be helpful in health terms, there is a real risk that research that only demonstrates probabilities for some people will be transformed into rules that apply in the same way to everyone, regardless of history or circumstance.

Like evidence-based decision-making, new technologies are offered as an unquestioned good; an unproblematic means of transforming primary care. They are presented as a means of ensuring continuity and of promoting shared service provision, with the only drawback being some technical issues surrounding the privacy of patient records. Privacy is indeed a crucial concern. We need strin-

Women and Health

"[There is a] considerable body of research, dating back to the early 1970s and continuing through the 1980s and 1990s, on the targeting of women in psychotropic drug advertising, and considerable evidence of harm to women from the overprescribing of benzodiazepines during the last 30 years."

Source: Barbara Mintzes, "Women and Drug Promotion: 'The Essence of Womanhood Is Now in Tablet Form,'" *Essential Drugs Monitor* (World Health Organization) 31 (2002), p. 13.

gent and enforced rules to prevent our electronic health records from falling into the hands of private health insurers or of employers. Both have strong incentives to avoid potentially unhealthy risks.

Important questions also arise about who puts the information into the records, about what kind of information is recorded, and about the rights that patients have to view, comment on, and remove information from their files. Women in particular have too often experienced diagnoses that reflect assumptions about women rather than appropriate assessments of their health problems, and such misdiagnosis can be perpetuated by these new schemes. These issues need to be resolved before too much information is recorded on a single file that is shared across services and providers.

Discussions on this front frequently imply that the new technologies can substitute for health personnel in providing continuity. Yet both within and outside institutions, continuous care from familiar personnel can be a critical aspect of effective treatment. Personal contact in care is decidedly important. A computer on the table cannot give you a warm smile or touch, nor does it engender much trust. Primary care reforms stress the importance of patients seeing the same physician, but do not place the same emphasis on seeing the same provider who is not a physician.

This tendency leads to the question of who provides the all-day, all-night primary care. One expectation is that nurse practitioners or other nurses will fill in during off-hours—an approach implying that care will differ depending on the time of day—or that telephone triage by nurses will help to fill the gaps. This approach creates a risk that, just as nurses might be substituted for physicians after hours, they might also be replaced by providers with less training and fewer skills. This situation already occurs in the United States, where "medical assistants" with very little training in health care staff many call centres for primary care organizations. Moreover, the goal in call centres can easily become keeping patients out of services rather than providing continuous care. Little evidence exists that such telephone services actually reduce emergency room use, although they may provide some needed comfort and advice.

Midwives

The gaps in primary care are linked to similar shortcomings in maternity care. Although care for pregnant women has been a part of public care since the beginning of publicly funded services, only a minority of jurisdictions offer full public coverage of midwifery care. The *Canada Health Act* makes no specific mention of midwives, although they could easily be understood to be one of the other health professions included.

In the distant past, many women in Canada relied on midwives during pregnancy and birth. But as a result of pressure from doctors concerned about the competition from midwives and questions of competency, the country made midwifery illegal. As early as 1865, Ontario medical men convinced the government to give them the exclusive right to attend childbirth. Women still practised legally long after that in some other provinces, but eventually the physicians won out everywhere in Canada. In making midwifery illegal, we got out of step with most of the world. Some women continued the practice, albeit in an underground network of care. In the 1960s midwives became increasingly popular amongst women seeking alternatives to what had become a medicalized hospital experience under physicians' control. It was not until twenty years later, however,

Midwifery Care in Canada: Barriers to Access					
Province	Legislated	Funded	Fee for Service	Practise Locations	Education Program
Alberta	Yes	No	Yes	Home/ Hospital/ Birth Centre	No
British Columbia	Yes	Yes	No	Home/ Hospital	Yes
Manitoba	Yes	Yes	No	Home/ Hospital	No
Newfoundland and Labrador	No	No	No	Hospital (re- mote areas only)	No
New Brunswick	No	No	No	Home	No
Northwest Territories	No	No	Yes	Home	No
Nova Scotia	No	No	Yes	Home	No
Nunavut	Partially (one pilot project in 2002)	Partially	No	Birth Centre (only on Rankin Inlet)	No
Ontario	Yes	Yes	No	Home/ Hospital	Yes
Prince Edward Island	No	No	Yes	Home	No
Quebec	Yes	Yes	No	Birth Centre	Yes
Saskatchewan	Yes	No	Yes	Home	No
Yukon	No	No	Yes	Home	No

Source: Miranda Hawkins and Sarah Knox "Midwifery Care Continues to Face Challenges: Canadian Midwifery Is Still Defining Itself, One Mother at a Time," *Canadian Women's Health Network* 6: 2/3 (Spring/Fall 2003).

that women saw some success in challenging the formal prohibitions against midwifery practice.

Despite their ancient history, midwives fit well with new approaches to health care. They take a health promotion approach to pregnancy and birth, rather than a narrowly medical one. Diet, exercise, and social relations are integral aspects of their care. The entire household can be involved, and every effort is made to put the women giving birth in charge of the process—which may take the form of birth at home rather than in a hospital delivery room, although midwives are usually prepared to assist in any location. Like some health reformers, midwives are firmly committed to continuity in care, ensuring that the same midwives accompany women through their entire pregnancy and beyond. Midwives begin their relationship with pregnant women shortly after conception and follow through long after birth. At the same time they are prepared to work not only in teams as midwives and with others in health services but also with families. They combine old approaches with new techniques. Not only that, they are less costly than doctors because they are paid less, they use less technology, and they do more preventative work that saves costs in the long run.

In the 1980s Ontario was the first province to legalize and pay for midwifery as part of the public system. Teams of midwives are salaried under the provincial health insurance plan. A midwifery program is offered at three Ontario universities, with Laurentian University offering courses in both English and French and adapting study to the particular needs of Aboriginal midwives. These courses ensure that midwives are appropriately educated both in the latest techniques for assisting before, during, and after birth, and in a philosophy of woman-centred care. The program includes an emphasis on cultural sensitivity in an effort to ensure that midwives can provide support in ways that respect the traditional cultural practices of the pregnant woman. Midwives can prescribe certain drugs and order particular tests, just as doctors can. They can work alone, or with doctors, in hospitals, homes, and birthing centres. In short, they can provide the kind of primary care that fits the definition developed by the World Health Organization. The main problem with care by midwives in Ontario is that there are not enough of them.

However, midwives are not generally understood as being covered by the *Canada Health Act*, and few discussions of primary care reform spend much time talking about them. No other province has gone as far as Ontario in terms of educating midwives and fully integrating them in the public health system. Instead, access to midwives depends entirely on which jurisdiction you live in. Newfoundland does not have any midwives, for example. Alberta allows them, but does not pay for them. As a result, midwives are not part of primary care teams in most of Canada, and they are not available to most Canadian women. Despite clear evidence that qualified midwives provide high-quality care and save money and despite the growing shortage of family physicians who provide maternity care, we have had little public discussion about making midwives integral to primary care reforms.

Primary Care Reform and Medicare

Primary health care is critical. Canadians need and want a primary care system that treats them as whole people with histories, families, and communities while providing continuity, health promotion, a range of providers, access and choice, and necessary equipment and services in ways that are accountable. However, in the name of choice, continuity, and health promotion, and against the backdrop of fiscal restraint, current proposals for primary care reform run the risk of significantly reducing choices for both patients and providers without clear evidence that the rostering and capitation strategies will either address the problems within the system or lead to better quality care. Pools of capitated, rostered patients fit well with U.S. models of Managed Care, but not with Canadian approaches to the funding of shared services. Given international pressures, they also set us up not only for U.S.-style health care but also for the provision of care by U.S. corporations.

Primary care reform is necessary and can be based on successful models already in place that address the well-known existing problems without incurring new risks. Several provinces have community health and special needs clinics funded with global budgets to serve specified populations. Patients are not required to enroll and may choose to make use of them for some but not all of the services they provide. These clinics are staffed with a broad range of providers, all of whom, including the physicians, are typically salaried. Elected community boards, as well as peers, usually set their broad policies. They can maintain effective links with other community services, and with hospitals, at least as well as can physician-based group practices, and they can enjoy the economies of scale to be able to introduce and operate new technologies where appropriate. Similarly, hospitals may provide primary care more effectively and efficiently in many locales. As several provider organizations in British Columbia suggested, the reform of primary care should not be based on a single approach. Instead, it should promote multiple models based on a core of shared principles.[8]

The reform package should include the further expansion of publicly funded midwifery. The presence of midwives enlarges the range of options available to pregnant women and reduces the pressure on family doctors. Midwives also contribute to improved primary care. They are available around the clock. They provide continuity of care, they emphasize education and social support, and they are ready to work collaboratively with other providers.

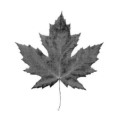

6. WHAT ARE THE
MAIN ISSUES TODAY?

Although the missing pieces and the details of primary care reform are critical to the system as well as to Canadians individually and collectively, they are seldom the stuff of headlines. Instead, wait times, labour shortages, and an aging population make the news—and are often represented as major problems that make the system financially and politically unsustainable. There is no question that these are all important issues. But whether they should be cause for panic and for the abandonment of our public system is by no means certain.

An Aging Population

More and more, the proliferation of aging baby boomers is used as a justification for panic about health care. All those babies born with the return of prosperity after the military came home from World War II are now growing old. According to those claiming crisis, too many old, sick people will be supported by too few young people. The assumption is that the elderly always cost the system more and contribute less than others.

This assumption can be easily challenged. Perhaps most importantly, age alone does not determine health-care costs. The last years or days of life are expensive in terms of care, but that is true regardless of age. Young people have serious accidents skiing or racing cars, too, and that could also be a major cause for concern when it comes to health-care costs. A young diver who has a swimming pool accident that leaves her confined to bed costs the system much more than a ninety-year-old who is simply frail. The care for a ninety-year-old woman is likely to become expensive when she comes close to dying, which could be at age one hundred.

We cannot base predictions about costs on the current elderly either. This aging generation is in much better health than the previous one was. They have grown up with public health care. Many have had decent, secure jobs and have pensions to support their health. They are also into keeping fit and eating properly. Of course, significant inequalities related to gender, racialization, geographical location, and class will play out even more in old age. Women live longer than men and have fewer economic resources to support them in their old age, for example.

Although some of the elderly will certainly need health care, we cannot assume that this will necessarily create an overwhelming burden, in part because other countries have been able to handle similar disproportionate populations without undue economic strain. In Japan, for example, more than one of five people is over age sixty-five, and in Germany 19 percent of the population is now in that age group. Canada is not projected to have 20 percent of its residents over sixty-five until the year 2024.[1]

Equally important, elderly people also pitch in to provide a great deal of care, especially if they are women. They care for children, neighbours, relatives, and spouses in ways that promote health and reduce overall costs to the system. In addition, they frequently offer financial support to their children in ways that keep those family members independent of government supports.

We do need to think about reforms to address the aging population. We need more specialists who understand the needs of the new elderly. We need better research on these needs. We need better prescribing practices, given that many of the health problems of the elderly result from medications. We need better attitudes towards the elderly, including more recognition of their contributions. What we do not need is to panic about an aging population in ways that justify more private care.

Wait Times

Wait times are our newest crisis. Not long ago we were phoned by a major Toronto newspaper asking for a horror story on wait times. When we offered a story about someone we knew who did not wait, we were told that was not news. What makes the news is a mother waiting in emergency for hours, or an elderly person left in a hospital hallway, huddled in one of those embarrassing gowns. What makes the news is a woman with breast cancer who cannot get radiation for a month, or a man in pain waiting for a new hip. In the wake of these stories and of people sharing real experiences, wait times have not surprisingly become a major preoccupation of both governments and the general public.

The Supreme Court decision on Chaoulli, which rejected the prohibition in Quebec against private insurance in areas covered by public care, centred on the matter of unreasonable wait times. The four judges who voted against Quebec's right to prohibit the sale of private insurance to cover services already covered under the public scheme based their arguments on a notion of freedom that emphasized an individual's freedom from government interference. In doing that they rejected a notion of shared rights to care gained through government intervention. The Court could simply have instead required the Quebec government to ensure reasonable access, thus upholding the collective right to determine services. As it turned out, the individual right to buy was reinforced. The decision opened a floodgate of demands for more private purchasing and for-profit delivery. Governments are paying even more attention to this issue, and those seeking to privatize both delivery and payment are moving in to take advantage.

CHA Principles Seen as "Handcuffs" by the Fraser Institute

For Michael Walker, the long-time head of the Fraser Institute, the famous five principles of the *Canada Health Act* are the "five handcuffs" constraining health care. The Institute's 1996 Five-Year Plan, "Towards the Next Millennium," declares its aim to "become Canada's leading source of information on private health care."

Source: *The Toronto Star,* March 25, 1997.

The Supreme Court decision reinforced the panic, but the issue was news long before that. Indeed, the 2004 federal/provincial/territorial agreement on new funding made reporting on wait times almost the only condition for new federal funding. After coming to office in early 2006, the minority federal Conservatives made wait times one of their five priority issues.

It was the Fraser Institute, a think tank supported by interests seeking privatization, that first made wait lists a crisis issue. It produced an annual series of studies claiming to reveal dramatic growth in wait times for surgery and tests in Canada. These studies were based on some doctors' opinions about wait times for elective surgery rather than on actual measures of wait times. The doctors said they thought wait times were growing and estimated how long people were waiting for specific kinds of care. The survey, then, was about opinions rather than about actual measures of how long people wait for care.

What do the actual measures show? Well, it depends on what we are measuring. Waiting for what—an appointment for an annual checkup, elective surgery, or emergency care? Waiting in each case can have very different consequences. Waiting in the doctor's office is more than annoying. It can mean loss of income for those paid by the hour or on piecework, and for those without paid sick leave, but it is not usually life-threatening. Waiting for cancer treatment may not be life-threatening either, according to the research, but with this terrible fear weighing on you, the wait itself may undermine your health. In assessing wait times, we not only need to know what people are waiting for but also what is an appropriate time to wait. We need to take into consideration the context of their lives and their physical and mental condition. We need evidence on how long is too long in terms of the impact on our health and the cost of treating everyone as soon as they seek care. These complex questions of measurement cannot be reduced to a simple story. The patient waiting for care in the Chaoulli case, for example, had already gone through multiple surgeries and was considered a high risk for further surgery. We need, then, to recognize that there can be other important reasons for waiting—reasons that have nothing to do with the availability of services.

Wait times are difficult to measure because it is also hard to tell when to start the clock. We may need time to decide whether we want the intervention or to organize our lives to have an intervention, especially if we are women who are responsible for the care of others. The patient in the Chaoulli case had taken himself off the waiting list at least once, which makes it difficult to determine exactly how long he had waited. Do we start when your knees first give you pain when you play tennis? Or when you first visit your family physician, or when you agree with your specialist on the decision to treat? How do we count the wait if, perhaps due to a cancellation, a patient is offered surgery three days later, as one of us once was, but has to turn it down because of another obligation—and in our case, a session on grant applications that same day? If I wait six months for an MRI because the doctor does not really think I need one, given that the X-ray already told us the source of the problem, should the wait be counted at all? These kinds of complex questions make accurate measurement difficult. We must also remember that the treatments themselves are not without risks, so it may be appropriate to refuse treatment altogether or for a doctor to put someone with a significantly better chance of survival higher on the list.

That many of the services and techniques being offered are quite new also has an impact on what seem to be increasing wait times. Popular interventions, such as knee and hip replacements, became widespread only quite recently, for example. It takes time for the medical establishment to learn how to do them well, to deal with the backlog of people who thought they would have to live with the pain, and to create the resources required to perform the surgery and provide the necessary physiotherapy.

The critics have also created the impression that people do not have to wait for such services in other countries. They create this impression in part by stories of people paying for quick care in the United States. However, the United States has no data on wait times for entire populations there, and even less evidence on which people wait. In assessing claims about wait times in the United States, we need to ask about how some people get fast service and about others who did not get any care at all. The data that do exist suggest that wait times in the United States are increasing, particularly in hospital emergency departments, and that many people never get on a waiting list at all.

We do have some data on wait times in Canada. We have these data in part because we have a public system that allows for some co-ordination and accountability. The federally funded Canadian Institute for Health Information (CIHI), unlike several provinces, counts wait times in terms of how long it takes from when the booking form is received until elective surgery happens. The resulting data do not suggest any reason for panic. According to that measure, CIHI reports that median wait times for non-emergency surgery remained virtually the same between 2001 and 2005.[2] At the same time, the number of surgeries increased enormously. In 2005–06, 42,000 more hip and knee, cataract, revascularization (heart), and cancer surgeries were performed in Canadian hospitals outside Quebec than were performed the year before. This represented a 7 percent increase in a single year, *after* adjusting for population growth and aging.[3] In other words, a lot more people had the surgery even though they did not have to wait longer than before. Meanwhile, Canadians do not wait long for emergency care. And we should also remember that we are frequently doing many surgeries now that a couple of decades ago were mainly experimental, so we have made significant progress within the public system. In short, the data do not suggest a crisis.

Equally important, the research indicates that a public system represents the best way of reducing wait times. There is no reason to assume that private payment and investor-owned service delivery will reduce wait lists. A lot of assumptions are made about for-profit delivery being better, but the clear evidence is that quality is lower

Long-Term Care

"We compared staffing levels of nursing and support staff... [in] 167 [B.C.] nursing homes, 109 (65%) were not-for-profit and 58 (35%) were for-profit.... The mean number of hours per resident-day was higher in the not-for-profit facilities than in the for-profit facilities for both direct-care (registered nurses, licensed practical nurses and resident care aides) and support staff housekeeping, dietary and laundry staff and for all facility levels of care. Compared with for-profit ownership, not-for-profit status was associated with an estimated 0.34 more hours per resident-day provided by direct-care staff... and 0.23 more hours per resident-day provided by support staff [both of which are statistically significant differences].... This finding suggests that public money used to provide care to frail elderly people purchases significantly fewer direct-care and support staff hours per resident-day in for-profit long-term care facilities than in not-for-profit facilities.... Although staffing differences do not necessarily imply differences in quality of care, an extensive body of research in the United States links higher direct-care staffing levels in long-term care facilities to better care outcomes."

Source: Margaret J. McGregor et al. "Staffing Levels in Not-for-Profit and For-Profit Long-Term Care Facilities: Does Type of Ownership Matter?" *Canadian Medical Association Journal* 172 (5), (March 1, 2005) <www.cmaj.ca/cgi/content/full/172/5/645> (Dec. 13, 2007).

and access more limited when care is provided on a for-profit basis.[4] In this regard we keep thinking about our recent experience with trying to set up our Internet connection with a for-profit firm. We spent longer on the phone trying to talk to a real person than we ever do when we call the doctor; and longer waiting to get an appointment with a technician than we do to see our doctor.

Alberta has just demonstrated that a public system can integrate resources in a manner that dramatically reduces wait times for knee and hip surgery. The province simply put the doctors and the tests in the same place, something a government is well placed to co-ordinate. The wait time to consult an orthopedic surgeon was cut from 35 weeks to 6, and the time from the consultation to the actual surgery was cut from 47 weeks to 4.7.[5] This means less private practice, rather than more, because it means doctors have to work together and with other services. Ontario demonstrated this long ago for heart surgery, when it developed a co-ordinated list throughout the province that also dramatically reduced wait times. As physician and health-policy expert Michael Rachlis says, specialized clinics and managed wait times in the public sector can provide superior service "while reducing overall administrative costs and providing broader societal benefits" such as equity.[6]

Adding private insurance, as the Supreme Court decision suggests, and adding investor-owned delivery services, as the Kirby report and others suggest, can only increase rather than decrease overall wait times. The system would become more fragmented and less co-ordinated. Some people would get faster care, on the basis of ability to pay; or the public purse would bear more of the expense. The result would not be more care but a shift in who gets care, and higher costs due to duplication and administration. We also know that private-sector services will not be readily available in rural areas or in low-populated regions because those places do not have enough people to allow private firms to make a profit. The private owners will not create more providers to deliver services but instead will reduce the number of providers available for public care. They will not relieve pressure on the public system, nor will they reduce costs. We know that they will increase inequality, because they operate within a system in which money will get people to the front of the line.

In a *New York Review of Books* article on the U.S. system, economists Paul Krugman and Robin Wells conclude that the U.S. approach brings with it high government costs, while "the actual delivery both of insurance and of care is undertaken by a crazy quilt of private insurers, for-profit hospitals, and other players who add cost without adding value."[7] Although privatizers and the Supreme Court claim that the model they advocate would be European rather than American, most of the firms seeking to take over delivery of Canadian care are based in the United States. Moreover, the trade rules, as well as many lobbyists, favour the U.S. way. Wait times have been a main lever in the movement towards for-profit insurance and care delivery.

Making wait times the crisis of the hour also distorts our priorities, as the Romanow Commission pointed out. The federal/provincial/territorial agreement in 2004 established five priority areas in terms of wait times: cardiac surgery and catheterization, cancer surgery, cataract surgery, hip and knee replacement, and MRI and CT imagery. These areas are now getting disproportionate attention and resources, leaving out the other health issues. Maternity care, for example, is not on the priority list even though a growing number of women are finding it difficult to find a care provider who will deal with this pressing health issue.

A focus on wait times can mean bad-quality care. In England, National Health Service hospitals are "having to repair damage done during botched operations on people who have been sent to private centres for hip and knee replacements to cut waiting lists." In two privately run centres where the figures were examined, the failure rates were significantly higher than in public hospitals—three times the rate in one, and ten times the rate in another. Training for surgeons was suffering, leaving a questionable future for quality care.[8]

There are certainly areas in which we need improvement. We need to better co-ordinate both administration and care. We also need to put more resources into care providers as opposed to technology and drugs. A major cause of waits for surgery and hospital beds, for example, is the failure to hire nurses full-time and to provide them with decent conditions for care. We need work not only on the practices, but also on the collection and analysis of data, as well as on the presentation of those data to the public. To address these needs, in 2005 the Liberal government under Paul Martin commissioned a report by a physician administrator, Brian Postl, on wait times. In addition to pointing out the problems with focusing on wait times alone, Postl also stressed the importance of producing better data. In particular, an appendix to his report clearly shows how the data on wait times need to take gender into account in assessing who waits how long for what care with what consequences. For example, women are twice as likely as men to suffer from osteoarthritis, the major factor in the need for hip replacement surgery, but no more likely to have the surgery.[9] This appendix makes the critical point that different populations have different needs as well as different access. It reveals how we have to examine the context of people's lives, taking social locations such as gender, age, racialization, sexuality, and physical ability into account in creating and analyzing the data.[10]

Although the evidence shows that wait times do not constitute a generalized crisis, and that privatization is not an appropriate solution to the problems that do exist, governments are being pressured to agree that a crisis exists and to move in the direction of privatization, even if by stealth. The Conservatives, along with other interests such as the Canadian Medical Association, are promoting wait-time guarantees as a way of saving the public system—but this approach has obscure, yet very real implications for privatization.

Wait-Time Guarantees

Wait-time guarantees appear to be a simple, attractive solution: a means of pressuring governments to reduce wait times and of ensuring that people have alternatives in care. The idea is that if a provincial medicare system is unable to make available a particular procedure within a pre-established and reasonable maximum time, it would guarantee to pay for this procedure in another province or in the United States, or from a private provider outside the provincial system. What is deemed "reasonable" would vary according to the specific procedure involved. It might be a certain number of months for a needed hip-replacement operation, and a certain number of days for chemotherapy to start after diagnosis or surgery for a specific form of cancer. Guarantees would be established for the large-volume procedures, including diagnostic procedures such as MRI and CT scans.

There are several reasons why we should not introduce wait-time guarantees, however. Focusing on guarantees for some services shifts resources away from other critical areas. Guaranteeing short waits for new hips could mean fewer operating rooms available for foot surgery or difficult births, for example. Guarantees can also mean shifting practitioners into areas in which they have little experience. It could also mean speeding up the care process. A doctor who usually does general surgery may be moved to knees and the person getting new knees, may be sent home much earlier. Research in the United Kingdom indicates that such practices have led to an increase in medical errors, and even deaths.

Guarantees can move resources around the health-care system in ways that threaten safety. In focusing on wait-time targets, U.K. hospitals have neglected cleaning in ways that have led to significant increases in deaths from superbugs. After all, guarantees move more care to the for-profit sector. In addition to allocating public money to profits rather than to care, this shift too puts patients at risk. Recent systematic surveys of research show clearly that for-profit care is not only lower in quality but also more dangerous than non-profit care.[11] Guarantees lock governments into focusing on current issues, leaving little room to respond quickly to new issues such as SARS and bird flu, or to some new, unexpected crisis. Ironically, given that doctors argue that a private system will reduce bureaucracy, wait-time guarantees would increase the need for bureaucracy because the government would have to monitor the private as well as the public system. Otherwise, how could we justify spending public money on private care if that private care was intended to ensure guarantees?

In short, some Canadians wait too long for some types of care, and continued efforts are vitally needed to improve the situation. Alberta, of all provinces, provides clear evidence that it is quite possible to address wait times effectively within the public system. We also have evidence that there are not large numbers of Canadians waiting too long for necessary care. The federal/provincial/territorial focus on wait times for cardiac surgery and catheterization, cancer surgery, cataract surgery, hip and knee replacement, and MRI and CT imagery has already started to produce reductions in wait times within the public system.[12] Instead of dealing with wait times by creating a legal and bureaucratic system of guarantees that concentrates only on selected conditions while increasing patient risk, we should follow the evidence by focusing on various aspects of the organization of public care, as Postl recommended in his recent report on wait times. These include improved benchmarks for reasonable wait times, more integrated wait lists, increased use of information technologies, better education for health professionals and the public alike, and the development of "surge capacity" to handle both unanticipated emergencies and planned events.[13]

Addressing wait times through care guarantees necessarily means more private care. Such care is often justified not only on the basis of care needs but also on the grounds that we already have private payment and some clinics. It is simply bad logic to say that we already have some private care and some people can now push to the front of the line, so therefore we should have more of both. It is like saying, "You already had some crime, so why not allow more?"

Costs and Sustainability

We have also heard repeatedly about how dramatically rising costs undermine government's capacity to develop other programs or even to continue with old ones. Was, or is, public health care the major cause of debts and deficits? Is it unsustainable for financial or other reasons? The answers to these questions are not simple, but they are not that public health care is unsustainable.

The major cutbacks in health-care expenditures that began in the 1980s were justified primarily in terms of excessive government spending and growing deficits. Prime Minister Brian Mulroney talked in the 1980s about the debt we were leaving our children. Newspapers were full of stories predicting a worldwide crisis resulting from excess spending on social programs. One report from New Zealand claimed that they had to shoot a hippopotamus because the public zoo could no longer afford to feed it. The story implied that we had to cut back on public services or risk extinction.

Writing at the time of the major panic about government deficits, two Canadian government economists, Hideo Mimoto and Phillip Cross, made the case that expenditures on social programs did not contribute significantly to the growth of the federal debt relative to the overall growth in the economy. Tax cuts were a much more important factor, reducing the size of the government pie and thus making the slice going to health care and other social programs look larger. Governments were also trying to fight inflation by keeping interest rates high. This too increased the debt by making government borrowing more expensive.[14]

In any case, while spending on health care has increased in Canada over the past thirty years on both a per capita basis and as a share of the GDP, as it has in every industrialized country, the rate of growth has been moderate since the introduction of medicare. More to the point, the private spending on health care has been growing more rapidly than has public spending. In 2002, the last year for which final figures are available, Canada stood eighth out of twenty-six industrialized countries in its public health-care spending as a share of GDP.

This distinction between public and private health-care spending is important. Too often, all health expenditures are lumped together, implying that they all come from the public purse. Yet it is by means of public payment that the costs can best be controlled. The modest growth in Canadian spending contrasts sharply with the continuing dramatic rise in the United States, where cost increases are arguably unsustainable. Over the three decades from 1975 to 2005, public spending on health care increased, on average, by 3.5 per cent annually, while private spending increased by 4.4 per cent. In recent years the gap has widened.[15] At about 7 percent, the shares of GDP devoted to total health-care spending were comparable in our two countries at a time when every province joined the medicare system in the early 1970s. The U.S. share is now over 15 percent, or half again as much as the Canadian share.

Meanwhile, whatever we don't pay publicly through taxes, we buy privately through insurance or directly over the counter, or we don't buy at all. If we buy privately, it is the sick and poor who pay

Health Expenditures by Source, Canada, 1975–2005			
Year	% Public	% Private	Total as % of GDP
1975	76.2	23.8	7.0
1985	75.5	24.5	8.2
1995	71.3	28.7	9.1
2005*	70.1	29.9	10.2

* Estimate

Source: CIHI, *National Health Expenditure Trends, 1975–2006*, Ottawa, 2006.

most, rather than the healthy and wealthy. If we cannot afford to buy privately, we do without, at least until our conditions become so unpalatable or dangerous to others that the state or charity kicks in.

Despite rounds of tax cuts, especially to corporate taxation, most governments in Canada have achieved balanced budgets or even surpluses. The federal government in particular has run substantial surpluses for close to a decade. Public debt is now well under control. We have the freedom to choose to spend more on health care, on other determinants of health, on the military, on further debt reduction, or on a combination of priorities. The choices are political. They are not forced on us by economic constraints.

Expenditures alone do not, then, justify the label "crisis." Nor do they justify a shift to private payment. Indeed, the highest-spending countries are the United States and Switzerland, the countries with the most private involvement. By 2005 total Canadian spending as a percentage of GDP had also fallen behind the levels in France, Germany, Austria, and even Portugal and Greece. We would argue that the time has come to spend relatively more, and to raise and spend the funds efficiently and equitably, through taxation.

Nevertheless, we cannot ignore the reality that public health-care costs have been rising—and would rise even more if we expanded the system to include at least home care, long-term care, and drugs. But if we are to assess both the possibilities for more care within the public system and the privatization alternative, we need to determine which costs have been rising most quickly.

Traditionally, at roughly 80 percent, labour costs have accounted for the lion's share of health spending. But while it would not seem unreasonable to focus on these expenditures, it would be a mistake to see unreasonable demands from labour as a primary cause of cost increases. According to the Canadian Institute for Health Information, "Census data show that, on average, employment incomes for full-time workers in health occupations rose at about the rate of inflation between 1995 and 2000. That compares to almost a

6% after-inflation increase for all earners."[16] In other words, health-care workers got less than their share, and their wages are not out of control.

Moreover, the incomes of health-care workers and their wage gains in recent years show huge disparities. Doctors are by far the highest paid members of the health-care sector, and their pay has continued to increase throughout the latest reform period. Unlike all full-time health-care workers taken together, the average pay, after expenses, of full-time doctors increased between 1995 and 2000 by 5 percent after inflation. Full-time specialists averaged over $140,000 in 2000, and family doctors over $120,000, while pharmacists averaged about $65,000. RNs and nurse supervisors averaged about $48,000, with RNAs just under $40,000 and midwives about $35,000.[17] Nevertheless, the proportion of total health spending going to doctors has been declining in recent years. This decline partly reflects efforts to reduce the increase in doctors' income through strategies such as maximums on the amounts they can bill in some areas and more surveillance of their billing. But it also reflects increased spending in other areas, notably drugs.

At the other end of the health-care income scale are those who are often called "ancillary" workers—the people who cook, clean, do laundry, serve food, and keep records. They are the lowest paid of all. These mainly female workers have been a primary target of cost-cutting in the form of contracting out services to the private sector. Eliminating jobs or reducing wages for the lowest paid workers saves much less money than would be saved by doing the same for managers or physicians. Yet this reality has not prevented ancillary workers from being targets for privatization. The small savings realized from this strategy come at a high price. A U.K. research study found that "the alleged savings" come with "unacknowledged and externalized costs" that are borne by patients "in terms of their health, the taxpayer in terms of the additional finance and cleaning staff in terms of job security, additional workloads and erosion of conditions."[18] The result of this strategy, then, has been job loss and deteriorating conditions for women as well as a decline in quality of care, at some risk to patients.[19] Nevertheless, our new public/private partnership hospitals in Ontario follow this model, defying the evidence.

If it is not the workers, what does account for the increase in costs? Again, much of the recent growth in health expenditures is attributable to drugs. More money goes to drugs than to doctors. New technologies, especially information technologies, also account for a significant share of these new costs. Despite all of the calls for accountability, the contributions of these technologies to expenditure growth are much more difficult to evaluate. Still, we do know that spending on information technologies, like spending on drugs, is growing rapidly even though there is often little evidence to show that certain technologies significantly improve patient care or increase efficiency.

According to an editorial in the *Journal of the American Medical Association*, "roughly 75% of all large IT projects in health care fail" and the problems are not "simply bits of bad programming or poor implementation."[20] When it comes to spending in this area we often operate on the basis of faith in technology, and the word of those selling it, rather than on the basis of rigorous evidence. We simply assume that more technology is better. With new information technologies, we lack even the limited safeguards that are in place for drugs. There are few requirements for demonstrating effectiveness before or even after purchase.

Both drugs and technologies are produced in the for-profit sector. In other words, the rapidly rising costs in health care come from the private for-profit sector even though the products involved have not necessarily been proven to be either efficient or effective in health-care terms. But these private interests, and in particular the drug industry, have been profitable. If we want to control costs, we should be targeting drugs and technologies rather than the services and the mainly female providers; and we should be extending public control over costs through means such as stronger drug regulation and bulk purchasing rather than moving to contract out services and build public/private partnerships. What is not sustainable is rapidly growing profits in health care and increases in for-profit delivery that allow public money to go to profit rather than care.

Another cost is also rising, but it is difficult to capture: the cost of all the reforms that have been happening across Canada. According to McGill University management professor Henry Mintzberg, "Government has, I think, gone overboard on outsourcing because of private-sector thinking." It has done that, for instance, by applying a narrow, readily measurable approach to "efficiency" that ignores unmeasurable benefits. Mintzberg cites the specific example of health care: "We're starting to find out what we lost, but it took years to find out. They knew what they were saving instantly. The loss of benefits took time to find out."[21] Nonetheless, governments and health service organizations have frequently followed this trend, at times even after business abandoned it.

Sometimes the cost of a reform is quite clear, though. When the provincial government amalgamated two Toronto hospitals, Sunnybrook and Women's College (along with the Orthopaedic and Arthritic Hospital), in the mid-1990s, the costs in signage and letterhead alone were surprisingly high. In 2006 the two hospitals were de-amalgamated, calling for new signs and new letterhead yet again. The money involved in these changes went to the for-profit sector when it could have gone to hire more nurses.

The supposedly cost-saving measure of amalgamating hospitals had another hidden cost: nurses had to be "let go"—and then nurses had to be sought out and rehired when nursing shortages became obvious. The practice of using employment agencies to replace nurses who are injured or ill as a result of working conditions or poor planning resulting from new managerial strategies creates another less visible, but nonetheless costly, expense.

In the health-care system as it is, a number of relatively simple steps, if taken, could save a great deal of money: avoid bad prescribing practices that result in thousands of hospital days each year;

Time to Take Superbugs Seriously

Sometimes a bit of alarm is a good thing. There is probably not enough alarm about the superbugs and other hospital-acquired infections that according to some estimates kill at least 8,000 people a year in Canada. That's as many as die annually in Canada from breast cancer (roughly 5,000) and motor-vehicle accidents (3,000). Imagine if 8,000 people died in the SARS pandemic of 2002–03 (just 44 did), from the West Nile virus (just two last year) or from AIDS (72). People would be terrified. They would demand that something be done.

Source: *The Globe and Mail,* Sept. 15, 2007, p. A24.

reduce medical errors through innovative programs that support whistle-blowers and prevent individual punishment while looking for collective solutions; keep health services clean so that patients and residents do not pick up superbug infections as a result of their unsafe environments; improve working conditions to reduce the injury and illness rates of health-care workers (rates that are more than double those in other industries); co-ordinate care in ways that reduce duplication. Those are just a few of the ways in which we could make the current system work better.

There is no shortage of ways to improve spending in health care, and the government coffers do have money that could go into this effort. Canadians have repeatedly shown in polls that they are willing to pay more taxes in return for better care. Instead of making cuts in the GST, for instance, government must respond by avoiding the cuts that force hospitals and schools to close. Again, as the Romanow Commission so clearly stated and substantiated, our public health-care system is as sustainable as we want it to be.

Labour Shortages

The media and researchers have identified another crisis area: a shortage of health-care providers. We hear constant talk about people without doctors, wait lines caused by nursing shortages, and therapies delayed due to lack of therapists. We are told that the crisis will only get worse because many of the practising doctors, nurses, and therapists are old and will soon retire. Moreover, more doctors today are women, and women will not put in the long hours that men do. To plan for care, and to participate in the discussion of ways to ensure that care will be there, we need to assess the extent of the shortage, its causes, and possible solutions.

Doctors

Canada does not have significantly fewer doctors per person than the United States does, and we have about the same number as the United Kingdom—though significantly fewer than the former Soviet Union and most of the countries of Western Europe.

The number of doctors per person in Canada has not changed much since 1990, and before that we had fewer doctors per person than we have now. What does distinguish us from the United States is the proportion of doctors who are specialists. In the United States 70 percent of the doctors are specialists; in Canada half of the doctors are general practitioners. Despite the stories about people without family doctors, 86 percent of Canadians can name their family physician. Still, for the 5 percent who cannot find a doctor (the other 9 percent report not looking for one),[22] the shortage is real. These people are more likely than other Canadian residents to live in rural Canada, to have recently moved to Canada or to a fast-growing location within Canada, or to be seeking a family doctor for the first time. Along with those who need care outside doctors' normal office hours, they may rely on hospital emergency rooms or walk-in clinics.

Neither Canada nor the United States has doctors evenly distributed in relation to the population. Significant provincial variations exist, along with significant variations within provinces, especially when it comes to specialists. Doctors are concentrated in large urban centres, where the teaching hospitals and medical schools are located. Physicians have free choice about their locations and face very few negative consequences for choosing a city over a rural area. Various strategies are being used to attract doctors to rural areas. Some municipalities are offering housing, special pay, and debt subsidies, or income guarantees. These are not strong incentives for Canadian medical graduates, however, given that they are virtually guaranteed not only employment but also high and secure incomes wherever they choose to locate. Some provinces actively recruit from abroad in an effort to overcome these obstacles, but recruiting from abroad is not without its problems. For one thing, these foreign recruits have been educated at their own countries' expense, and their own countries need them. For another, there is no guarantee that they are any more likely to remain in rural areas for long. In fact, they may have even more motivation than the Canadian-born to leave rural areas because they can find more compatriots in major urban areas. Then, too, in 2004 22 percent of our doctors became MDs outside Canada. This figure represented a decline from the 1970s, when the figure was about 30 percent.[23]

The province of Ontario has undertaken a promising strategy for attracting doctors to rural areas. Learning from an Australian model, in 2004 the province established a medical school in the North. To gain admission applicants must demonstrate a strong commitment to the North, and much of their training takes place in small, remote communities. That work includes their entire third year, which is spent with a group of physicians in one such community. Their fourth year is spent at regional hospitals in Thunder Bay and Sudbury. The hope is that, after receiving their education in small and large communities in the North, they will form social and professional ties or maintain old ones that will keep them there. Special efforts are being made to recruit Aboriginal people and to ensure that the education that all recruits get is culturally sensitive. Not incidentally, this new school was the first to be built in many years, and it signals a new government investment in the physician labour force.

Although we are not now suffering from major shortages in urban areas, it is the case that we may face shortages in the future. It would be overly simplistic to assert that this situation follows from years of reductions in the number of medical school spaces. These reductions resulted, in part at least, from a recommendation that researchers made to shift some care away from doctors to other practitioners. The researchers showed that most health-care costs were the result of doctors' orders and that doctors were both the most expensive health-care providers and the ones trained to do the most expensive interventions. The researchers argued that shifting more care to other providers such as nurse practitioners and other health-team members would directly reduce costs: more care would be provided by those who are paid less and indirectly, and the number of expensive interventions would be reduced through preventative work. Unfortunately, the number of doctors educated was reduced without the accompanying recommended changes, so we do not know if the advice was appropriate or not. In any case, we have been graduating fewer doctors relative to the population. Ontario has begun work towards increased enrollments in medical schools, not only in the new Northern school but also in the old ones. Other provinces are doing the same. Across Canada the absolute number of physician graduates started to increase in 2002, after a small dip in the mid-1990s.

There has been a dramatic change in the doctor population that we are graduating. While women were a tiny minority of physicians and surgeons until universities were pressured to alter their admission practices in the 1960s, they are now a majority of those enrolled in medical school. They are still a minority of practising physicians, but this will soon change—which is good news for Canada, because women are more willing to be family physicians and to work in clinics or group practice. It also means that more women seeking medical care can see a women doctor if they prefer. Moreover, women are more likely to be tied by family to remaining in Canada. It is the case that female doctors tend to work fewer hours than their male counterparts do, in large measure because they still retain primary responsibility for children, families, and household work. But more male doctors too are seeking a life outside work, one that includes their children. Younger male doctors too are working fewer hours than are their more senior colleagues. It is only reasonable that doctors work hours similar to those of others in the labour force, and to plan accordingly.

The entry of women into medicine may slow as tuition rises, in part because women earn less than men and thus have less to put into their tuition. For the same reasons, entry may slow as well for the students from immigrant and racialized communities who have been entering medicine in significant numbers. For all these groups, the lengthening of medical education may also have a dampening effect on future enrollment. The longer time spent in medical school has contributed more to the doctor shortage that we now face than has the reduction in the number of spaces in these schools.

Almost all of our doctors do stay in Canada. Some—and in particular young specialists—go to the United States, seeking greener pastures, but many return after they discover that they have more autonomy in our public system than they do in the largely insurance-controlled U.S. system. Indeed, the latest CIHI figures indicate that more doctors are returning than leaving. It is nevertheless important to develop strategies to keep them here, not only because we need them but also because we have invested heavily in their education. We could make them pay back at least some of that investment before they leave, and we could educate them better about the U.S. system.

Doctors are protected through their powerful professional organizations. They have been able to successfully resist many reform initiatives, including attempts to put them on salaries. Some younger specialists may be tempted to leave, and doctors' organizations have maintained their members' right to locate wherever they choose. There are, however, signs from the organizations of medical students and of medical interns and residents that many of the young doctors

In 2004, out of a total of about 62,000 practising physicians in Canada, 262 picked up stakes and moved outside the country—but in the same year 317 physicians returned.

Source: CIHI, *Health Care in Canada* 2006, Ottawa, p. 23.

support public care. More are willing to work in group practices and clinics, where they will have support from colleagues. As a result, more may be willing to work in non-urban areas. This tendency may bode well for the future in terms of supply.

If we are to deal with the shortages that do exist, we need more ways of ensuring equal distribution of doctors. We do need to educate more doctors, but we also need to change how they practise if we are to ensure a sufficient supply.

Nurses

Nurses form the single largest occupational category in health care. They make up just under half of all health professionals, and more than nine out of ten of them are women. The female dominance is important because it remains a factor in their more limited power. It is a factor as well in their efforts to distinguish themselves through an identification with science rather than their old association with traditional female skills.

Nurses fall into a number of different categories. Nurse practitioners, whose numbers are tiny but growing, have gone in and out of fashion in Canada. These nurses with additional education are now being promoted as a means of both emphasizing prevention and of reducing the reliance on doctor care. They are a cheaper alternative and can deal with many of the issues that doctors now handle. Still, not many patients can be shifted to their care because there are still fewer than one thousand of them across the country. However, given that not all of these nurses are working to their full capacity, there is room for improvement even with these numbers. In

Registered Personnel in Selected Health Professions, Canada, 1998–2006						
	1998	2002	2006	% change 1998–2006	Per 100,000 pop., 1998	per 100,000 pop., 2006
Physicians[1]	56,163	59,412	62,307	11	186	190
Midwives[1]	265	413	622	135	0.9	2
LPNs	73,751	60,123	67,300	NC	245	205
RNs[2]	233,336	236,094	257,999	11	774	787

1.   Includes individuals not currently employed in the profession.
2.   Includes Registered Psychiatric Nurses, excludes Nurse Practitioners.
NC   data not comparable.

Source: CIHI, *Number of Health Personnel in Selected Health Professions, by Registration Status, 2006*, Ottawa, 2007, and calculations by authors.

summer 2007 Canada's first nurse-practitioner-led clinic opened in Sudbury. Funded by the provincial government, it provides patients with the opportunity to receive the full range of services for which nurse practitioners are trained. The nurses at this clinic work in partnership with, but not under the direction of, family physicians.[24]

The largest nurse category is the registered nurse. Now educated in universities, RNs are critical to institutional and community care. In fact, the delays in emergency caused by people waiting to get into a hospital bed are most commonly caused by a lack of nurses. The same is true of surgery. Much of the public discussion about a nursing shortage is related to the age of this category of nurses. A majority of these nurses are now at least forty-five, and well over a third are at least fifty. Many are near retirement or looking forward to it soon.

Licensed practical nurses (LPNs), also called registered nursing assistants or registered practical nurses, constitute another major nursing category and another essential component in care. They too are aging. Like the RNs, the overwhelming majority of LPNs are women, although there are relatively more men doing this kind of nursing work. This group also has more women defined as visible minority. A significant number of those working as RNs and LPNs have been recruited from abroad, which raises the same questions that arise for doctors. The issues, and thus the solutions to the looming shortage, are much more complicated than an aging labour force.

Many qualified nurses are not working full-time in their profession. Some work part-time because they are women with household and unpaid care responsibilities. Some use casual work as a means of juggling demands. But the main reason is that employers are not offering full-time permanent jobs, even as they complain about current and pending shortages. This tendency is in turn partly related to government cutbacks and the lack of stable funding. During the reforms of the 1990s the closure of hospitals and other health-care facilities meant layoffs for thousands of nurses. Many went to the United States and remain there. Mike Harris, the premier of Ontario at the time, proudly announced that nurses were going the way of hula hoops; out of fashion and out of use.

The shortage is also related to the adoption of for-profit management techniques. Nurses are made to work harder and faster, with fewer others around to help. "Just enough nursing," as defined by managers, is too often not enough. Nurses struggle to make up the care deficit. As a result, their injury and illness rates have soared well above the rates for police officers or construction workers, who receive much more attention in that regard. In fact, nurses face more violence on a daily basis than do the police. This too reflects cutbacks that prevent them from providing the care that people need and that they want to deliver. The work is becoming more demanding just as the labour force becomes older. Under such conditions it is not surprising that many want to leave the profession and that younger nurses are not staying in the work as long. Solving the nursing shortage, then, requires much more than educating more nurses or recruiting more from abroad. It means changing the conditions and relations at work.

Obviously, the way in which employers manage the number of nurses available on any shift is an important factor in how hard nurses have to work. Less obviously, the number of nurses who are working permanently together also makes a difference. It takes time for new nurses or nurses who are casually employed to learn specific routines, and it uses up the time of other nurses as they learn. Least obvious in discussions of the working conditions faced by nurses, at least in public media, is the nature of their teamwork with the ancillary workers. The employees who cook and feed patients, who clean floors and laundry, who keep records and transport patients: these workers are doing jobs once done by nurses. It is essential work that must be done. When it is done by those trained for the work, it leaves more time for nurses to do other aspects of their job. Ancillary workers also help to ensure a safe environment for nursing work. In recent years, however, this work too has been significantly cut back. Compared to nurses, ancillary workers have faced even more managerial reforms designed to control their work and reduce staff to an absolute minimum. More ancillary work is being done by those not trained for the job. More of it is being done by outside contractors. Research on cleaning services in British Columbia shows that when the work is contracted out, not only does the quality decline but nurses also spend more time getting the cleaning work done.[25] In other words, cutbacks in other areas and changing managerial practices increase the pressure on nurses and their workload.

Most nurses are organized into unions or professional organizations. Starting in the 1960s, these organizations were successful in transforming what was understood as a labour of love for women, to be done without much financial reward, into work with decent pay and benefits. But the organizations did not have enough power to resist the reforms based on arguments that both deficits and rational planning justified transformation. In recent years, nurses' organizations have marshalled their strength. They have demonstrated through research the critical link between good working conditions for nurses and good care.[26] They have also effectively used the shortage issue to win new hires, more permanent positions, and better conditions.

Nurses and their organizations are generally supported by the public. Nevertheless, there is still a way to go before we can speak of good conditions for nursing care. Those who do ancillary work have been less successful in defending their employment or conditions of work. Although a significant proportion were unionized, contracting out has reduced the number who have union protections in part because the skills and contributions of these mainly female workers are less visible.

The nursing shortage is as much the result, then, of nursing conditions as it is of a lack of trained personnel. We have a shortage of those willing and able to work in health care or willing and able to stay there. Solving the problem thus requires paying attention to these conditions, as well as to the education of new recruits.

Other Health-Care Workers

Other areas of health care also have shortages of workers. In radiation therapy, for example, governments cut back on the number of places in the education system. Combined with deteriorating working conditions, this decrease in supply has contributed to the wait times for cancer care. As is the case with nurses, the solution requires more than training. It also involves addressing the conditions of work.

In other words, there is no reason to panic about labour shortages in health care. We do not have a significant overall shortage of doctors right now. It is more a problem of distribution and of specialists in a few areas. With so many doctors due to retire, we do need to admit more doctors to medical schools. We are beginning to do that and more. The new Northern school is a fine example of how governments can work to address shortages. Nor do we have a shortage of nurses. Rather we have a shortage of good nursing jobs. We need to educate more nurses, but this approach will not do us much good unless we also change their conditions and relations of work. Finally, we need to train and maintain the full range of employees in health care. Ancillary workers are as critical to care as are other providers, and they play important roles in health care. Shortages here, of jobs if not of available workers, may well be as significant as shortages of doctors and nurses.

The issues raised about wait times, costs, and labour shortages, although meriting discussion, do not, then, constitute a crisis in the system. The questions surrounding these issues can be solved within a public system. Indeed, the record shows that a public system is the only place in which they can be solved effectively, efficiently, and equitably.

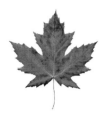

7. PUBLIC STRATEGIES
AND SHARED SOLUTIONS

The language of crisis so prevalent today is being used mainly to justify a single strategy for change: privatization. After a relatively quiet beginning, out of the public eye—in part because our system has so much popular support—privatization has taken on a more visible face. Still, much of the push and many of the changes are going on below the surface of public debate, making it critical for all Canadians to recognize the signs and understand the consequences.

At the same time a number of other effective reforms are being introduced across Canada that can serve for models elsewhere, and some old practices are worthy of maintaining and copying. These examples tend to be much less dramatic and much less visible than are the stories of crisis. They are nonetheless alternatives to privatization that should be at the centre of the public discussion.

Privatization

Our health-care system has always had its private elements. When medicare was introduced, it was designed as a public insurance scheme that differed significantly from private insurance. There was no assessment of our health before we joined. All of us were eligible, and there was no maximum on the care received and no co-payments for services. We paid for the health-care system through taxes without regard for our health status, even in those provinces that used the label health premiums for some of their taxes. Equally important, we had full choice about what services we used and when we used them. It was, nevertheless, public payment for private practices and services.

Initially at least, medicare mainly meant that governments paid for existing services rather than providing these services directly. Most doctors were, and remain, in solo or group practices, working in their own offices. Most of them rely on the fees negotiated with their provincial governments. They make comfortable incomes, but very few are in the business of making profits for shareholders. Most hospitals are also private in the sense that they are not owned by the governments that pay for hospital services. Almost all of them, though, are not-for profit or charitable organizations and are heavily regulated by government. Until quite recently, management in these organizations was dominated by those with medical training. Some costs have also long been paid by individuals and their families or by insurance companies. A great deal of care has long been provided by friends and relatives, most of them women. In short, certain parts of the system are private in terms of ownership, payment, and responsibility.

Forms of Privatization

Increasingly, more and more aspects of the system are being privatized. Here we are using privatization in the broadest sense to refer to the shift away from health care understood as a collective responsibility for a human right—with care based on need and provided in the spirit of public service—to health care understood as a consumer good and a private responsibility—with care based on ability to pay and provided in line with business principles. The nature and extent of privatization vary considerably across the country. There are, nevertheless, common patterns that result from global pressures and agreements as well as from local government initiatives and local issues. These common patterns of privatization take a number of overlapping forms that have an impact on cost, quality, equity, and democracy. While few of these forms are entirely new, together they constitute a qualitative shift away from public care—and they make a major departure from the approaches that we have traditionally experienced under medicare.

Private payment for health care is one form that privatization takes. Expenditures on health care are rising throughout the world for many reasons. Medical advances, which mean that more can be done than in the past, and demographic pressures contribute to increased spending. But other factors include the increasing extraction of profits, the fragmentation of complex systems, and ill health caused by poverty and poor working conditions. One way in which governments have been responding to increased costs is to shift responsibility for payment to others. This form of privatization is justified not only in terms of saving the government money, but also as a means of preventing the abuse of what are often regarded as free services. The assumption is that we value what we pay for directly and will think twice about using services if we have to pay.

Although the *Canada Health Act* prohibits fees and extra-billing for hospital and doctor services, governments have found other ways of making people or their insurance companies pay for care. The act does not define "medically necessary," which opens the way for governments to "delist" services that they will no long cover. This has happened with eye exams and in vitro fertilization, for example. Removing people from hospitals, or preventing them from going there, has the same effect because outside the hospital, fees and even charges for the total cost of care may apply. Less visible is the privatization of costs that result from governments failing to create needed services as new health issues emerge. Treatment for Aboriginal peoples with AIDS is one example that emerged in the international conference on HIV/AIDS held in Toronto in 2006. Even less visible is the shift in other costs involved in moving to home care.

At home the costs of extra laundry, special food, and cleaning, as well as equipment and medicine, are increasingly borne by the private household.

Yet there is little evidence to suggest that these moves to more private payment relieve the economic pressures on governments. Among ten leading industrialized countries in 2003, only Norway spent more per capita from the public purse on health care than did the United States. Canada ranked seventh, slightly behind France, Germany, Sweden, and Switzerland (another country highly reliant on private payment), and slightly ahead of the United Kingdom, Australia, and Japan.[1] Private payment has not reduced the expenditures of these countries—which is not surprising given that fees and payments cost money to collect and these costs can outweigh the amounts collected. It also costs money to sort the deserving from the undeserving, as the Hall Commission recognized long ago. For people with limited resources, even the smallest fee can prevent them from seeking care. They thus forgo necessary care, often creating significantly higher costs in the long run. If diabetes is not detected because annual checkups are no longer without charge, the cost of caring for the effects of untreated diabetes can be much greater for governments than is the money gained from limits on care. For those with ample resources, fees have little influence on their use of the system and thus cannot prevent abuse. Meanwhile, the need for the collection of such fees makes the system needlessly complex. In addition, physicians determine almost all hospital and prescription drug use, and fees for patients do little to change their practices. One group of researchers called user fees "zombies"—they are ideas killed by the evidence long ago, but keep being raised from the dead.[2] Nevertheless, fees can mean extra income for the individuals who charge them, which helps to explain their persistent resurrection; and they seem to make sense if you do not look at the evidence. Moreover, they have an obvious appeal to those who feel they can afford to pay or who believe strongly in the sanctity of individual choice.

For Profit Facilities—Low Quality and Deadly

Most evidence examining for-profit healthcare comes from the United States, where there is a mix of private for-profit, private non-profit, and public hospitals. And that evidence is overwhelmingly in favour of not-for-profit healthcare…. A recent review of 149 studies and 20 years' worth of data looked at how these facilities performed… in the areas of access, quality, and cost-effectiveness…. The researchers looked at six types of institutions—hospitals, nursing homes, HMOs, hospices, dialysis centres, and psychiatric hospitals. They found that 88 of the studies concluded that non-profit centres performed better, while 43 studies found that the performance was no different. Only 18 studies found for-profit centres were better. The differences are particularly clear at psychiatric inpatient hospitals, where out of 17 studies, only one found for-profit facilities to be better…. Tragically, a recent systematic review that followed 500,000 dialysis patients for a year showed patients receiving treatment in for-profit centres are significantly more likely to die than those treated in non-profit ones: expanded to all Americans who receive dialysis, this means as many as 2,500 premature deaths every year may be due to being treated at for-profit centres.

Source: Canadian Health Services Research Foundation, *Mythbusters*, "Myth: For-Profit Ownership of Facilities Would Lead to a More Efficient Healthcare System," revised and updated, March 2004 <www.chsrf.ca/mythbusters/index_e.php> (Nov. 15, 2007).

Considerable evidence indicates that private payment increases inequality in access to care. When governments do not pay, or when they charge fees, individuals either pay directly for the service, buy insurance to cover the service, or go without care. Women have fewer economic resources than men do and less control over economic resources. Women are also less likely than men are to have insurance coverage through paid work; they are less likely to be able to pay the fees or buy insurance. Women are thus more likely than men to go without necessary care. Moreover, because significant differences exist among women in access to economic resources, the shift to private payment leads to increasing differences among women in access to care. The same principle applies to anyone with limited resources. When access is based on ability to pay, inequality necessarily results even with very small fees. Although private payment is often presented as a way of allowing individual choice, it denies that choice to people who don't have the means to pay. It establishes choice only for those with the means to pay.

The privatization of care delivery is another common form that it takes. Given that most services have never been under the direct ownership of government, this form of privatization typically does not involve a move from government to private ownership but rather a move from private non-profit to private for-profit ownership. These different uses for the term "private delivery" can lead to confusion, which in turn often obscures the major impact of the move to for-profit ownership of care delivery. The confusion allows those promoting such privatization to argue that Canadians care only about who pays for their services and not about who delivers them. The move is justified on the grounds that the private sector will be more efficient, effective, and responsive, and that the private sector has more resources. Increasingly, these privatized services are also promoted as a means of taking the pressure off the public system and of reducing wait times for care.

The public debate has been largely about the establishment of for-profit clinics to deliver outpatient surgical services. Several provinces now allow these clinics (Ontario, for one, has prevented the establishment of for-profit medical clinics). Considerable debate also surrounds the advent of public-private partnerships, or P3s, involving hospitals. British Columbia and Ontario, for example, have launched several P3 hospital projects. A for-profit consortium builds the hospital; it designs, finances, and manages it; and it operates some or all of its cleaning, laundry, food, maintenance, clerical, laboratory, and security services. The P3 model builds on the practice, found in most provinces, of contracting out cleaning, laundry, and food services within non-profit institutions, but P3 arrangements are locked in for much longer periods.

Here, too, little evidence supports the claim that for-profit organizations are more efficient and effective at delivering care. But significant evidence does indicate that costs are higher and capacity and service are reduced, and thus quality may well be lowered.[3] Indeed, as U.K. research shows, governments often spend more when for-profit organizations deliver care. According to Frank Dobson, formerly the senior U.K. health minister, private firms earn 11 percent more than the U.K.'s public National Health Service for delivering the same procedure. Another estimate puts the gap at 40 percent. Part of the reason is that the for-profit sector is granted a higher fee schedule to entice it to participate. For-profit firms also typically negotiate for a fixed level of activity, which eliminates their risk in the process. The risk is transferred to the public purse, which pays for the process in full whether or not the negotiated level is reached. As a result, some family doctors have reportedly been "bribed" to direct their patients to for-profit facilities.[4]

New drugs and technologies can produce some savings in health care. Thanks to new drugs, some patients can be safely discharged more quickly from expensive hospital stays, and new information and organizational technologies can on occasion give rise to genuine efficiencies. But the implementation of these reforms is at least as easy to introduce in the non-profit sector as it is in the for-profit sector, and the for-profit sector has no more control over the prices of drugs and technologies than does the non-profit sector. Indeed, those prices can sometimes be driven down through bulk purchasing by governments, regional health authorities, and consortia of provider institutions.

Most of the costs in health care—between 70 percent and 90 percent, depending on the service—are labour costs. Thus the main way in which for-profit companies can save money in providing care is through reducing labour costs. They lower labour costs by hiring fewer providers, by making each of those who remain work faster and longer and by paying them less. For-profit firms also tend to employ providers with less formal training at lower costs.

Because women are the majority of paid providers, they are the ones who most often see their care work transformed in ways that often threaten their conditions of work, along with their health. More of the jobs are now part-time and casual; more of those doing the work are defined as self-employed. Job security disappears for many, while others simply lose their jobs. For nurses, privatization often means working for a for-profit, temporary help agency that charges facilities more for their services than regular employees would cost. Or it may mean working for a for-profit home-care service that does not hire anyone full-time. In both cases the nurses are less likely than other nurses to have union protection. As a result, they are less likely to have protection for pay, vacations, and conditions of work, and from harassment in all its forms.

Most frequently contracted out is the cooking, cleaning, and laundry work. This work has traditionally been defined not only as women's work but also as unskilled work and thus as worthy of less pay. In British Columbia, contracting out or outsourcing this work has meant job losses for 10,000 unionized workers. It has also meant foreign ownership of the services, leaving Canadians with less control over conditions of work. Those who kept their jobs saw their wages cut almost in half. Their benefits were either eliminated or drastically reduced, and the guarantees of work hours and job security abolished.[5] The conditions of contracting often ensure this is the case. Moreover, contracting out pits worker against worker because those working within the same institution have different employers and different conditions of work. The majority of these workers are women, and a disproportionate number are immigrant women and from racialized groups. As a result, inequality is further reinforced. Significantly, though, in June 2007 the Supreme Court struck down as unconstitutional three sections of British Columbia's 2002 legislation that had invalidated important provisions of the collective agreements then in place. The provincial government was given twelve months to pass new legislation respecting the collective bargaining process in the areas of contracting out, layoffs, and "bumping" (or seniority provisions for employment security).

The deterioration of working conditions in health care reverberates throughout the economy, contributing to low wages for women in other sectors. Equally important, in health care the quality of working conditions shapes the quality of care. Poor working conditions make for poor care. As the quality of care declines as a result of work reorganization, the mainly female patients suffer.

Private delivery inevitably costs more because after the workers, supplies, buildings, and equipment are paid for, the company also has to make a profit. For-profit organizations, unlike non-profit ones, have to have money above and beyond what goes to care—that is their very reason for being. For-profit firms also have to pay more to borrow money to finance capital projects. Governments can borrow at lower interest rates. With the financing of P3 projects by the private sector, governments can appear not to have incurred additional public debt, but in the long run the drain on the public purse is greater because of the higher interest charges involved.

For-profit firms are interested only in those parts of health care that can be delivered quickly, that can bring big and fast returns in assembly-line fashion. Private clinics want to work only on medical procedures that deliver the most lucrative returns on investment. They specialize in areas that are subject to quick intervention, and they often use techniques developed in the public system. For example, in cataract surgery, a profitable line of work, important surgical procedures were developed by researchers employed in a non-profit Ottawa hospital. Now for-profit clinics offer this surgery, claiming that their innovative practices deserve just rewards. These clinics operate in several provinces, with the public purse often meeting the costs of their services. Yet there is no reason why the public sector cannot operate such clinics on a non-profit basis. Indeed, they already do. Toronto's Orthopedic and Arthritic Centre, for example, which is now part of a large, multi-site hospital, specializes in a limited range of surgical and rehabilitation services. After more than half a century of pioneering in its field it remains fully integrated within the public system.

If anything goes wrong in a private clinic, or if a case is complicated in any way, the patient and the costs are shifted to the public system. The for-profit sector thus "cherry picks," taking the easiest cases while leaving the rest, the more complex, along with their medical failures, to a public system that necessarily becomes more costly as a result. Governments also have to step in when companies close due to bankruptcy or when they are no longer making what they consider to be a reasonable profit. Governments cannot allow the only hospital in town to close, and they cannot easily replace it with a more competitive one.

The delivery form of privatization is, not surprisingly, particularly popular with firms seeking profit, because it gives them the best of both worlds. Governments guarantee both payments and profits. This solution is especially promoted for wait-time guarantees, with for-profit firms providing, at public expense, services that are not available within designated waiting periods from non-profit providers. The promoters of these guarantees, such as the Harper federal government, argue that as for-profit firms invest in promising ventures, the result will be increased resources available for health care. But the promoters fail to mention that they cannot create more of the most critical resources in health care: doctors, nurses, and other health professionals. We have only a finite number of these professionals. If they work in the private system, they cannot work in the public one. If doctors are allowed to work in both, they place themselves in a clear conflict of interest. As research on eye surgery in Alberta has shown, doctors who work in both systems bring patients in the public door but offer them faster private service and longer wait times for public care.

Another, and directly related, form of privatization comes in the shift to for-profit methods of delivering services *even within* the public and non-profit sector. Traditionally health care has been defined as a commitment to care, guided by evidence on treatment and cure rather than by business practices. But now business practices are increasingly being embraced within and among public and non-profit organizations. The language of this "bottom-line" approach is the language of business, with services marketed to consumers and customers, with business plans and business strategies, with CEOs and product lines. It may be "business-like," but it typically lacks the practical, efficient, and effective qualities that this term suggests.

Management grows, as does information technology, in order to more closely control those actually providing the care. Meanwhile, the ranks of the care providers are thinned, at least relative to growth in the populations they serve and in the complexity of the proce-dures they perform. Purchaser/provider splits proliferate, diverting resources from care to endless cycles of writing and scanning for "requests for proposals," or RFPs to deliver services, preparing and evaluating the subsequent proposals, signing the contracts, and re-porting on and monitoring the actual service delivery. Parallel sets of lawyers, accountants, and bookkeepers are employed by both the purchasers and the providers. Meanwhile, different contracts go to different suppliers, making both service integration for the system and continuity of care for the care recipient more difficult to achieve. "Transaction costs," or the administrative costs associated with being business-like, rise; the quality of care stagnates or even declines.

Numerous examples refute the assumption that for-profit meth-ods are more efficient. Research shows, for example, that the costs of heart surgery in the United States, where much of the surgery is performed in for-profit hospitals, are on average double what they are in Canada, with mortality outcomes for patients that are no bet-ter.[6] When Manitoba experimented with the privatization of some home-care services, citizens' concerns resulted in a close assessment of the experiment. The province found for-profit delivery to be more expensive and lower in quality, prompting it to return to public de-livery.[7] A group of Toronto hospitals had a similar experience with for-profit housekeeping services, with a similar outcome.

Another faulty assumption is that health-care services are like any other business. But health care is a distinct form of service, quite different from McDonald's or Wal-Mart. Perhaps most obviously, health care is about life and death; about healthy possibilities and dangerous consequences. Delivering poor quality care carries risks, and both skilled work and working conditions are more important factors than in other sectors. Health care treats people at their most vulnerable in environments that constitute a high risk. It is also much less predictable than the rush at lunch for McDonald's. You may be able to ask a patient who needs to drop off a blood specimen for a lab test to take a number, but you cannot ask a woman about to give birth to do so.

Privatization methods have been most clearly applied to the major cost in health care: the cost of labour. As is the case in the for-profit sector, time-motion studies are used to reorganize, control, and speed up the work, leaving health-care workers in the public system, according to those we have interviewed, "with no time to care" and "not enough hands."[8] Members of the mainly female labour force feel guilty about the quality of care they provide, and often put in unpaid overtime to make up for the care deficit. Patients see and feel the speed-up that is defined as efficiency. The patients feel guilty as well when they ask for care. In the process, health care has become our most dangerous industry, with health-sector workers over 50 percent more likely than other workers to miss work due to illness or injury. And such figures underestimate the numbers who are made sick or injured at work on a daily basis. Our survey of workers in long-term care indicates that nine out of ten had suffered work-related job-time loss over the last five years.[9] These violence and other health issues add to the overall cost of care, while undermining quality and worker morale.

For-profit methods have also been applied to the overall organization of the system. In Ontario the government dramatically reduced the number of hospital beds and closed whole institutions based on the assumption that hospitals should run at 95 percent capacity, just like hotels. The 2006 terrorist attacks on the subway

Privatization of Home Care, Manitoba-Style

Home-care services were contracted out on a limited basis in Winnipeg in 1997. Very early in this "experiment," the provincial minister of health backed down from claims that the approach would improve quality of care and bring the promised savings of $10 million a year. Indeed, as it turned out, neither savings nor any improvement in quality occurred. It also came to light that Olsten, the U.S.-based multinational contractor, had a dubious record in its home country. It was, at the time, and had been in the past, the subject of a number of criminal investigations for false billings, failure to carry out the plan of care, and overselling services to vulnerable patients. Because all of these past actions had been settled out of court, Olsten was able to say that it had never been convicted.

Sources: CCPA-MB, *The State of Public Services in Manitoba: Privatization — The Public Service Trojan Horse*, Winnipeg, 2007; and Jim Silver, *The Cost of Privatization: Olsten Corporation and the Crisis in American For-Profit Home Care* (Winnipeg: CCPA-MB, 2000).

and bus systems in London and the 2003 SARS outbreak in Toronto show that you cannot run hospitals at 95 percent capacity because you always need surge capacity to respond to an emergency or even the daily variations in illness. This form of privatization too can be challenged on the basis of the evidence.

The privatization of care work by sending it into the private household represents another of these overlapping forms. With the dramatic expansion of public health systems following World War II, paid health-care work expanded enormously, especially for women, and the resulting rise in costs became a justification for cutting back on formal care. But it would be a mistake to see unreasonable demands from the mainly female labour as a primary cause of cost increases. The largest wage gains did not usually go to women, and, when they did, they merely meant decent wages for highly skilled work. In any case, wage gains in recent years have been lower in health care than elsewhere. Another justification for sending care work home is often taken from the women's health movement itself, which has at times been one voice among many maintaining that institutional care is bad for our health and that people want to be cared for at home.

Increasingly, this work is being sent home to be done by women or expected of women, even when their relatives and friends are in institutional care. It is characterized as sending care *back* home, implying that women have shirked their traditional duties there. But there is nothing natural, traditional, or unskilled about cleaning catheters, applying oxygen masks, and dressing wounds. Despite talk about returning care to the home, most of this new care work was not traditionally done there, and there is no evidence that the care that was provided at home in the past was all good care.[10]

That reality does not, however, prevent women from being blamed for not providing care, nor does it prevent them from feeling guilty when they are unable to meet care needs. It also does not protect their health or their paid work while they provide care. A Decima Research Survey of unpaid providers found that half of them had difficulties with their emotional and physical health as a result of care work.[11] Some 70 percent said that "providing this care had been stressful." Not surprisingly, those with both eldercare and child-care responsibilities, most of them women, are the most likely to lose time at their paid jobs as a result of caregiving.[12] This form of caregiving thus has social as well as economic costs in both days lost at paid work and declining social networks. Men are also not entirely protected from such work. Increasingly, men too are left to take on more home-care work when services are reduced and no women are around to do the work.

The shift to care in the home ignores another factor: many people do not have homes, or homes appropriate for care. Many homes are socially inappropriate, characterized by violence or other social conditions that prohibit or threaten care. Moreover, the shift of care to households increases inequality among women, because economic resources that allow women to hire others are unevenly distributed, and so too are relatives and others who can help with care. This form of privatization, then, hurts us all, but it has a particularly harmful impact on women in ways that increase inequality among them as well as for them.

In another form, the privatization of responsibility, we are increasingly held to account for our own health by both the dominant media and the reorganization of health care. The shift in responsibility for health to individuals and families, away from governments, is evident in the strategies to reduce hospital stays and institutional care of any form. It is evident in the stress on individual prevention and lifestyle as well. It is particularly evident in the focus on obesity. Again it is mainly women who are held responsible for their children's health and that of their partners, although we are all targets in this campaign.

This form of privatization is often presented as a response to demands for empowerment and health promotion, and there is some justification for this claim. We do need more of both. Yet the move to this kind of privatization ignores how structures of inequality and power undermine our possibilities both for taking responsibility and for shaping health conditions. An Aboriginal man living in the North, for example, pays extraordinary prices for the poor-quality food that is shipped there during a time when he and his people have found it increasingly difficult to follow traditional eating patterns. Eating poorly can hardly be blamed on that man. This form of privatization contributes to an overall shift in ideology, one that undermines our sense of both collective responsibility and collective risk.

Yet another form of privatization relates to decision-making. As more care is delivered by private and foreign corporations, fewer of the decisions are open to public scrutiny and influence. More of the decisions are based on money and made by those with money. As care is reorganized, more of the decisions about how long and how much care is provided are taken out of the hands of patients and providers, most of whom are women. If doctors are allowed to work in both the private and public systems, as some of them are demanding, even more of the decision-making will be in their hands and in the hands of those who can pay for care.

Privatization is not one process, then, but many. It is about a shift in who provides care, in who pays for care, in how care is provided and where it is provided, and in who is responsible and who decides. It is a fundamentally gendered process because women provide most of the care and use services in specific ways, although they often have little control over the structure of health care. Given the structure of its labour force, health care is classed and racialized as well. The specifics differ across the country but many of the processes and outcomes are the same. Access to care and conditions for care work are deteriorating, while inequality and costs increase. Yet privatization is still offered, and even implemented, as the main response to a highly touted crisis in care.

Where to Go from Here

We need to shift the debate from a perception of crisis to a focus on strengths. We know the strengths in a public system. The onus should be on those who want to privatize delivery and payment to show how investor-owned services and private payment will maintain or improve on these advantages. The public system offers a long list of established advantages. Those who want to privatize payment and delivery should be required to address these advantages when they seek to justify their claims.

That quality of care is higher in the public system is a result, in part at least, of having the rich use the same services as the poor. The rich thus have an interest in making sure that these services in common are good. If the bed you use today was used by a homeless man yesterday, you want to make sure he had a good and clean bed. It is also a result of governments maintaining uniformly high standards that are not easy to enforce in for-profit enterprises. In health care, it is difficult for the individuals using the system to judge what care is effective and whether quality is high. Care is not like buying shoes or a video game. We need intervention and assessment from experts in the field, and we are getting that through government organizations such as Ontario's Institute for Clinical Evaluative Sciences and Manitoba's Centre for Health Policy, which help to establish practice guidelines based on the best available evidence.

Questions for the Privatizers

Quality is not easy to measure, but we do have a host of studies indicating that quality is likely to be higher in public and in non-profit settings than in for-profit ones.[13] The question privatizers must answer is, "How will the quality be maintained or improved?"

The administrative costs are lower in a public system. Much less money is spent sorting the deserving from the undeserving or on denying care, as a U.S. colleague put it. Less is spent on billing and on chasing those who have not paid.[14] The question for privatizers is, "How will administrative advantages be maintained or improved?"

In a public system the central planning of the distribution of services makes it possible to more fairly distribute services across the country, and especially in rural and remote areas. In our medicare system, while we clearly have not been entirely successful, in part because we have left many of the decisions up to private organizations and individual doctors, we have reached many people who had not been reached before. The question for privatizers is, "How will the distribution of services be maintained or improved, especially for those outside of the urban core?"

In a public system wait lists can be centrally managed to allow an efficient and needs-based distribution of services. The examples of heart surgery in Ontario and joint replacement surgery in Alberta demonstrate this, and more public initiatives are underway. The question for privatizers is, "How will the advantages of these wait lists be maintained or improved, and how will we ensure that those most in need get priority?"

The central planning of a public system can also reduce wasteful duplication of services. For-profit systems assume duplication. Otherwise there is no competition to bring down prices—the competition that, according to free-market supporters, creates private-sector efficiency. The question for privatizers is, "How can we ensure that money and resources are not wasted on advertising, excess capacity, and other unnecessary expenses found in investor-driven systems?"

In a public system, where access is based on need rather than on ability to pay, the result is both more equity and more efficiency. Health care can be allocated to the sick and injured, rather than to the worried well. The question for privatizers is, "How will we ensure that equitable access and efficiency are maintained or improved?"

Jobs are better in the public sector, especially for the overwhelmingly female labour force that does the ancillary work. We know that better jobs translate into healthier workers as well as better care. The question for privatizers is, "How would employers be able to resist the pressure to cover increased private health insurance, and what would happen to industrial relations, labour-market efficiency, and the health of Canadians to the extent that employers are successful in resisting?"

Employers save significant amounts of money with a public system. They don't have to contribute heavily to employer-based health insurance, which means their costs are lower. This benefit is particularly important for long-established employers with lots of retired workers. With a public system, the risks and costs are shared among all of us. This benefit is particularly important for people who experience catastrophic illness or injury costs, and for a smoothly operating labour market in which workers can take or leave jobs without concern for the health insurance benefits attached to them. The question for privatizers is, "How will employers maintain their competitive advantage, benefit from or even avoid the pressure to cover more private care?"

Innovation on a large scale has been possible in the public system. Insulin, penicillin, the polio vaccine and anti-malaria drugs, for example, were developed in the public realm. As a result, we have had wide access to these products and processes. The question for privatizers is, "How will innovation of this fundamental sort be supported or enhanced, and how will those innovations be shared?"

Now costs are controlled through government budgets. The question for privatizers is, "How will costs be controlled? What happens when complications arise in the private system, when there are cost overruns, when people trained mainly with public money seek to work only in private care while reducing resources in the public system? What happens when health-care businesses fail or when people are refused care in the private, for-profit system?"

A public system makes collective, democratic decision-making possible, even if such decision-making is not always practised or available. We must also ask, "How will citizens, who contribute to all health-care services, directly and indirectly, have their voices heard in the design of health services? Especially the employed poor without the means to access private care? Who will decide—the patient with the money or the doctor with the expert knowledge, or citizens together? How will we maintain a balance between collective and individual rights? Who will decide how much money goes to profits rather than to care?"

Although some aspects of care will remain private, we need to collectively decide how the line should be drawn in relation both to the demonstrated advantages of the public system and to our notions of social justice. We need to figure out how that line can be drawn in ways that are based on evidence, widespread accepted principles, and public participation, rather than on the basis of power and ability to pay.

Increasingly, we are told, by the Supreme Court among others, that everyone is doing it. All the countries similar to ours are turning to the private sector. Actually, some governments and health-care organizations are turning back to the public and non-profit sectors, despite the active promotion of privatization by international agencies such as the Organization for Economic Cooperation and

Development, World Trade Organization, World Economic Forum, and their local allies. But even if the trend happens to be more towards privatization than away from it, should we simply embrace what is fashionable? We never allowed our children to use that argument and see no reason to accept it here. Let's instead look at the evidence for equity, access, effectiveness, efficiency, quality, and democracy. It tells us not to go the private way.

Other Means: Big Ones

The means of maintaining, sustaining, and improving public care have already been identified by various public investigations that have marshalled the evidence and consulted a wide range of Canadians. Achieving these goals requires political will on the part of the federal government, the kind of political will that brought us medicare in the face of strong opposition. The opposition comes not only from the big provinces but also from forces such as doctors' organizations and those even more powerful forces seeking profit. These means also require provinces and territories to think and work in terms of the country as a whole, and in terms of a future beyond the next election. They require an informed public willing to demand the kind of public care that Canadians have indicated again and again that we want.

What this means in practice is sustainable funding at the federal level, provided on the basis of enforced principles of the sort set out in the *Canada Health Act*. In 2004 the federal government committed an additional $41 billion over ten years to the provinces and territories for health care. If the inflation rate remains low, if governments spend the extra funds wisely, and if demands for introducing new technologies and new drugs are not excessively expensive, the funds should go a long way to keeping the public system, as we now know it, financially sustainable. The federal government will, however, have to show much more willingness to enforce the *Canada Health Act* provisions, and the provinces and territories will, for their part, have to commit more resolutely to the long-term, stable funding of their existing medicare services.

Maintaining and sustaining medicare also require an expansion of the national plan to include home care, long-term care, dental and eye care, and pharmacare throughout the country. All provinces provide some funding for these services, but the coverage is uneven. To have an effective return on the provinces' investment while ensuring equity and efficiency, we need national standards and systematic funding. Hall made this clear long ago, and his arguments remain relevant. Romanow recommended such an expansion, but followed the strategy used for doctor and hospital care: to begin only with some parts. The lesson from that strategy was growing public support resulting from the increase in access, efficiency, and effectiveness. The other important lesson, though, is that it is too easy to be stalled at this stage of the reform and move no farther. In the process efficiency is lost because various players work the system in ways that do not encourage the allocation of patients to the most appropriate level of care. Instead, they are sent to the funded level. We need, then, the full range of necessary services in each of these areas, and we need them without the complicated fee structures and eligibility rules that serve to increase costs while denying access to care.

Co-ordination of care in ways ensuring that people receive care in a timely fashion, according to appropriate standards, does not mean uniformity or a lack of choice. Indeed, we need a variety of services and approaches that allow us to respond to the diverse needs of our population. This is also the case in primary care. These services and approaches need to be linked in ways that avoid needless duplication and ensure quality care.

In health care the quality of working conditions is related to the quality of the services provided. We need national registries to allow us to ensure that providers are appropriately educated and to allow better distribution of the health-care labour force, but we also need to have national standards to ensure decent conditions of work. The

Canada Health Act says that doctors, dentists, and others working in hospitals should be reasonably compensated. This principle should hold for all those involved in care services. We also need adequate numbers of the full range of health-care workers to ensure both quality care and the retention of workers.

In all of this, too, we need public accountability. This means much more than counting services, inputs, and outcomes. It means more than patient satisfaction and health status surveys. It means as well more collective decision-making and ways of ensuring that politicians keep their promises to defend public care. This, in turn, means a reversal of privatization because privatization in all its forms means more private decision-making, as well as lower quality, less accessible, more expensive care.

Other Means: Little Ones

The necessary strategies all require major federal or provincial initiatives. There are, however, many smaller projects that serve as models for good public care. Some were in place long before medicare. Others are very recent. What they share is a demonstrated effectiveness in providing for care and a non-profit approach to care.

Michael Rachlis brings together many of these models in his books *Strong Medicine* and *Prescription for Excellence*.[15] One of his main points is the need to make health care safer by ensuring clean environments, good food, and careful prescribing. New palliative care units focused on care over treatment are another feature that he promotes as a model that saves money while improving quality. Ways of managing chronic diseases have been developed that take a proactive and co-ordinated approach that improves health and independent living. There are also a host of strategies for prevention, all the way from safer sidewalks, which help prevent enormous costs in broken hips, to getting the lead out of our environments, to restricting pesticides and herbicides that cause cancer.

We have many models of community clinics that have worked

well for years. They have community boards to make overall policy decisions. They have a salaried, interdisciplinary workforce that provides integrated and continuing primary care. They range in styles from the women's health clinic in Winnipeg that serves a specific population, and the Sault Ste. Marie community health centre that helps its patients avoid needing hospital care, to the community clinics set up under the initial Quebec health plan. Quebec's CLSCs have social workers and pharmacists, doctors and therapists, all working together to provide primary care and to link with home-care services and hospital services.

We know how to make medicare work better. We have plenty of models to follow. Many of these would save money, even in the short term. What we need is the political will and the ability to resist the forces for privatization.

Health Care and Social Justice

Our health system does have its problems associated with rising costs, deteriorating working conditions, aging populations, and wait times. We need to address these real issues, and others, collectively, while recognizing their impact on individuals. But the problems do not constitute a crisis in the public system. They are no cause for panic. We can address them without dismantling the system or starting from scratch. As we've seen, they are best solved within a public system.

The headlines themselves are creating a crisis because the representations of crisis are being used as a means of undermining faith in the public system and of justifying privatization. There are critical implications of framing the various problems as crises. We have to ask who benefits from reforms and who loses. We cannot ignore the profits now being made, and to be made, in health care in areas formerly covered by governments and not-for-profit organizations. Nor can we ignore the profits to be made, and now being made, from government-funded care. We have plenty of evidence of the pressure from the health-care lobbies and of the profits to be made in health care.

Health care is fundamentally about social justice, about our commitments to each other, and about collective rights and responsibilities. The struggle over reform is a struggle over what form of justice will prevail, over whether solidarity, community, equity, compassion, and efficiency defined in terms of public good will take precedence over individual rights to sell, purchase, and consume based on market principles and profits. It is a struggle over power and equity. As Roy Romanow said in the introduction to his report on the future of health care in Canada—a report he called *Building on Values*—the health-care debate is fundamentally about values.

Health-care reform is also about evidence. We are talking about a material world in which we have developed adequate means of assessing reforms in terms of quality, access, equity, and cost-effectiveness. In other words, the debate is not simply about my good versus your good. It is also about what we know about what works for whom in what ways. The assessments that have been done provide solid evidence that we can use as a basis of our values debate. It is often hard to sort the evidence from the values, partly because they are integrally related. But we do have good research, developed from a variety of sources and perspectives, that provides a firm basis for policy development and change. Unfortunately, as Krugman and Wells put it in their article on U.S. health care, "The bad news is that Washington currently seems incapable of accepting what the evidence on health care says."[16] We could say the same about Ottawa, Toronto, Edmonton, and Quebec City.

The debate over health-care reform is further complicated because our health-care system is complicated, because similar reforms are often put forward by both those promoting social justice and those promoting profits, because reforms frequently have contradictory consequences, and because we are all so individually and personally involved in health care. Recent articles in Canadian newspapers on access to new and expensive drugs, for instance, attack the public system as being coldly bureaucratic for denying "life-saving care." But those drugs may not in fact represent any advance over existing drugs. In the Chaoulli decision the Supreme Court used the Morgentaler case on access to abortion as a basis for supporting individual rights to private health insurance. Discussions about what is private and what is public in health care are often confusing. Such complications make democratic decision-making more difficult to maintain.

That is why all Canadians need to become informed participants in the health-care debate. We need, as informed participants, to work to ensure that governments at all levels take the responsibility for ensuring the right to care rather than shifting responsibility, as they have been in recent health-care reforms. The evidence clearly indicates that a public system offers the only possibility for collective, democratic decision-making. A strong public health system begins by recognizing that health care is a human right and that governments have a central role to play in ensuring the right to care. The right to care means access based on need rather than on ability to pay or on employment. A strong public health system means establishing the working conditions under which it is possible to provide the care that people need. It means recognizing that we have shared risks and shared responsibilities.[17]

Taking responsibility does not necessarily mean that governments must directly provide all the care that people need or even indirectly provide all the care desired. Nor does a public system necessarily guarantee democratic decision-making. But it does mean ensuring that access is not based on ability to pay. It thus means reducing or eliminating private payment for necessary care. It also means regulating the conditions of work to ensure both appropriate working conditions and quality in care, including care in the household. It means creating the structures for community participation in decision-making about health services and promoting genuine transparency in decision-making. In turn, this means reducing the role of for-profit methods and delivery. At the same time it involves providing a range of services, including institutional facilities, that offer alternatives to home-based care and that offer supports to those who provide care in the home, including support to continue in or return to paid employment.

While the impact of health-care reforms on women is both greater and more negative, many men too face deteriorating conditions for care with privatization. The deterioration is also greater for those who lack resources and face other forms of discrimination, such as immigrants, racialized groups, and the elderly. As the labour force becomes feminized in the sense that more jobs are like traditional women's work, and as more care is sent home, more men are facing precarious employment and reduced access to care; and more men are expected to provide care. As more access is based on ability to pay and as more care work is distributed on the basis of ability to purchase it, inequality increases among the entire population.

Someone must pay for and provide care. Sharing both the costs and the responsibilities is the only equitable approach to care. In assessing and planning for health-care reform, we must also ask the value question: What about equity, power, quality, and care? Only a public system can hope to meet the criteria of access, equity, quality, and cost-effectiveness based on democratic decision-making about care. Private solutions will leave too many of us waiting for care. Resisting privatization effectively while continuing to improve our valued medicare system requires us to arm ourselves with the evidence on health-care structures and reforms. It means creating the tools and structures for our meaningful participation in collective decision-making about public care.

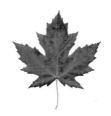

WHAT YOU CAN DO

1. Join your local health coalition. You can find information about this on the website for the Canadian Health Coalition, a not-for-profit, non-partisan organization dedicated to protecting and expanding Canada's public health system for the benefit of all Canadians. The CHC was founded in 1979 at the Canadian Labour Congress-sponsored S.O.S. Medicare conference attended by Tommy Douglas, Justice Emmett Hall, and Monique Bégin. The coalition includes organizations representing seniors, women, churches, nurses, health-care workers, and anti-poverty activists from across Canada. See its website: <www.healthcoalition.ca>.

2. Join the Council of Canadians. Founded in 1985, the Council of Canadians is Canada's largest citizens' organization, with members and chapters across the country. According to its website, the Council members work "to protect Canadian independence by promoting progressive policies on fair trade, clean water, energy security, public health care, and other issues of social and economic concern to Canadians. We develop creative campaigns to put some of the country's most important issues into the spotlight. We work with a network of over 70 volunteer chapters to organize speaking tours, days of action, conferences and demonstrations. We also produce research

reports, create popular materials, and work with individuals and organizations across the country and around the world. We do all of this to ensure that governments know the kind of Canada we want." Visit its website: <www.canadians.org>.

3. Run for the board of your local hospital or community health centre.

4. Visit the office of your local member of Parliament or of the provincial legislature and ask how you can work for public health care. Become involved in election campaigns, or even run yourself.

5. Join a union working on medicare issues. The website for the Canadian Labour Congress, the organization that brings together unions across Canada, offers a good entry point. See its website: <www.canadianlabour.ca>.

6. Keep informed by regularly visiting websites of all of these organizations and others, such as the Canadian Women's Health Network: <www.cwhn.ca>.

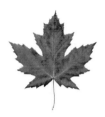

ENDNOTES

Chapter 2: How Did We Get Here?

1. Leonard Marsh, *Report on Social Security for Canada* (Toronto: University of Toronto Press, 1975 [1943]).

2. David Naylor, *Private Practice, Public Payment: Canadian Medicine and the Politics of Health Insurance 1911–1966* (Montreal and Kingston: McGill-Queen's University Press, 1986).

3. Dennis Gruending, *Emmett Hall: Establishment Radical,* revised ed. (Markham: Fitzhenry & Whiteside, 2005), p. 111.

4. Canada, *Report of the Royal Commission on Health Services* [Hall Royal Commission] (Ottawa: Queen's Printer, 1964); Canada, *Canada's National-Provincial Health Program for the 1980s: A Commitment for Renewal* [Hall Report] (Ottawa: Health and Welfare Canada, 1980); Canada, National Forum on Health, *Canada Health Action: Building on the Legacy. The Final Report* (Ottawa, 1997); Canada, *Building on Values: Report of the Commission on the Future of Health Care in Canada* [Romanow Commission] (Ottawa, 2002).

5. Canada, Senate Committee on Social Affairs, Science and Technology, *The Health of Canadians—The Federal Role. Final Report, vol. 6, Recommendations for Reform* [Kirby Report] (Ottawa: Parliament of Canada, 2002).

6. Antonia Maioni, *Parting at the Crossroads: The Emergence of Health Insurance in the United States and Canada* (Princeton, NJ: Princeton University Press, 1998).

7. Carolyn Tuohy, *Accidental Logics: The Dynamics of Change in the Health Care Arena in the United States, Britain and Canada* (New York: Oxford University Press, 1999).

Chapter 3: What Did We Get?

1.   Philip E. Enterline et al. "Effects of 'Free' Medical Care on Medical Practice: The Quebec Experience," *New England Journal of Medicine* 288:2 (31 May 1973).

2.   David Himmelstein et al., *Bleeding the Patient: The Consequences of Corporate Health Care* (Monroe, ME: Common Courage Press, 2001), p. 191.

3.   *Eldridge v. British Columbia (Attorney General)* [1997] 3 S.C.R. 624.

Chapter 4: What We Did Not Get

1.   S. Woolhandler et al., "Costs of Health Care Administration in the United States and Canada," *New England Journal of Medicine* 349 (2003), pp. 768–75; Himmelstein et al., *Bleeding the Patient.*

2.   National Forum on Health, *Canada Health Action: Building on the Legacy, vol. 2, Synthesis Reports and Issues Papers* (Ottawa: Minister of Public Works and Government Services, 1997), "Values Working Group Synthesis Report," p. 19.

3.   M. Hollander and A. Tessaro, *Evaluation of the Maintenance and Preventive Function of Home Care* (Ottawa: Home Care/Pharmaceuticals Division, Policy and Communication Branch, Health Canada, 2001).

4.   CIHI, *National Health Expenditure Trends, 1975–2006* (Ottawa, 2006), Figure 39, citing *OECD Health Data 2006.*

5.   Joel Lexchin, "Income Class and Pharmaceutical Expenditures in Canada: 1964–1990," *Canadian Journal of Public Health* 87:1 (1996), pp. 46–50.

6.   R. Tamblyn et al., "Adverse Events Associated with Prescription Drug Cost-Sharing among Poor and Elderly Persons," *Journal of the American Medical Association* 285:4 (2001), pp. 421–29.

7.   See, for example, Joel Lexchin, *Transparency in Drug Regulation: Mirage or Oasis?* (Ottawa: Canadian Centre for Policy Alternatives, 2004); Barbara Mintzes, *Drug Regulatory Failure in Canada: The Case of Diane-35* (Toronto: Women and Health Protection, 2004 <http://www.whp-apsf.ca/en/index.html>.

8.   Joel Lexchin, *Canadian Drug Prices and Expenditures* (Ottawa: Canadian Centre for Policy Alternatives, 2007), p. 14.

9.   Marcia Angell, "Excess in the Pharmaceutical Industry," *Canadian Medical Association Journal* 171:12 (December 7, 2004), p. 1451. See also Angell, *The Truth About the Drug Companies: How They Deceive Us and What To Do*

About It (New York: Random House, 2004).

10. Angell, "Excess in the Pharmaceutical Industry," p. 1452.

11. Stephen G. Morgan et al., "Whither Seniors' Pharmacare: Lessons from (and for) Canada," *Health Affairs* 22:3 (May/June 2003), p. 52.

12. Lisa Priest, "The Killing Cost of Drug Treatment," *Globe and Mail*, November 20, 2006.

13. Megan E. Coombs et al., "Who's the Fairest of Them All? Which Provincial Pharmacare Model Would Best Protect Canadians against Catastrophic Drug Costs?" *Longwoods Review* 2:3 (2004), pp. 13–26.

14. Alan Cassels, "National Pharmaceutical Strategy's Progress Comes under Scrutiny," *Canadian Medical Association Journal* 175:10 (November 7, 2006), p. 1194.

15. Margaret J. McGregor et al., "Staffing Levels in Not-for-Profit and For-Profit Long-Term Care Facilities: Does Type of Ownership Matter?" *Canadian Medical Association Journal* 172:5 (March 1, 2005), pp. 645–49.

16. See, for example, Dennis Raphael, ed., *Social Determinants of Health: Canadian Perspectives* (Toronto: Canadian Scholars' Press, 2004).

17. R.G. Wilkinson, *Unequal Societies: The Afflictions of Inequality* (New York: Routledge. 2001).

18. "The Social Determinants of Health: An Overview of the Implications for Policy and the Role of the Health Sector," an overview of a conference, "Social Determinants of Health Across the Life-Span," held at York University, 2002 < http://www.phac-aspc.gc.ca/ph-sp/phdd/overview_implications/01_overview.html>. Quote from L. McIntyre, G. Walsh, and S.K. Connor, "A Follow-up Study of Child Hunger in Canada," working paper W-01-1-2E, Applied Research Branch, Strategic Policy, Ottawa, Human Resources Development Canada, June 2001.

Chapter Five: Reforming Primary Care

1. World Health Organization, "Alma Ata Declaration," 1978, quoted in Julia Abelson and Brian Hutchison, "Primary Health Care Delivery Models: What Can Ontario Learn from Other Jurisdictions?" a review of the literature submitted to the Ontario Ministry of Health, April 1994, p. 3.

2. See, for example, Walter Rosser and Ian Kasperski, "Organizing Primary Care for an Integrated System," *Healthcare Papers* 1:1 (Winter 1999), pp. 5–22; Ontario, HRSC, "Primary Health Care Strategy"; Miles Kilshaw,

"A Strategic Plan for the Reorganization of Primary Care and the Introduction of Population-Based Funding," a report presented to the Federal/Provincial/Territorial Ministers of Health, 1995.

3. Rosser and Kasperski, "Organizing Primary Care," p. 12.

4. For an elaboration of one such proposal, see Milliman and Robertson, "Proposed Inter-Professional Primary Health Care Groups (PCGs) Costing Models," a technical costing report prepared by the accounting firm Milliman and Robertson for the HSRC's "Primary Health Care Strategy," 1999.

5. Rosser and Kasperski, "Organizing Primary Care," p. 14.

6. Rosser and Kasperski, "Organizing Primary Care," p. 9, estimate 90 percent of Ontarians can do so. Hugh Skully, "Building on One of the Best Delivery Systems in the World," *Healthcare Papers* 1:1 (Winter 1999), p. 27, reports that 81 percent of Canadians consider themselves to have a regular doctor.

7. Milliman and Robertson, "Proposed Inter-Professional Primary Health Care Groups," p. 5. Indeed, some U.S. health maintenance organizations do just this, ignoring that the studies leading to this guideline were conducted on men only.

8. B.C. Nurses' Union, Hospital Employees Union, and B.C. Government and Service Employees' Union, "Blended Care: Blending the Best of Institutional and Community Care, Making the Most of the Health Care Team," Vancouver, 1999.

Chapter Six: What Are the Main Issues Today?

1. Statistics Canada, *Portrait of the Canadian Population in 2006, by Age and Sex, 2006 Census* (Ottawa: Minister of Industry, 2007), p. 9.

2. CIHI, *Waiting for Health Care in Canada: What We Know and What We Don't Know* (Ottawa, 2006), p. 29.

3. CIHI, *Health Care in Canada 2007* (Ottawa, 2007), p. 28.

4. See, for example, Charlene Harrington et al., "Does Investor Ownership of Nursing Homes Compromise the Quality of Care?" *American Journal of Public* Health 91 (2001), pp. 1452–45; P.J. Devereaux et al., "A Systematic Review and Meta-Analysis of Studies Comparing Mortality Rates of Private For-Profit and Private Not-for-Profit Hospitals," *Canadian Medical Association Journal* 166:11 (May 28, 2002), pp. 1399–1406; Devereaux et al., "Comparison of Mortality between Private For-Profit and Private Not-for-Profit Hemodialysis Centers: A Systematic Review and Meta-

Analysis," *Journal of the American Medical Association* 288:19 (2002), pp. 2449–57; Devereaux et al., "Payments for Care at Private For-Profit and Private Not-for-Profit Hospitals: A Systematic Review and Meta-Analysis," *Canadian Medical Association Journal* 170:12 (June 8, 2004), pp. 1817–24; Steffie Woolhandler and David U. Himmelstein, "The High Costs of For-Profit Care," *Canadian Medical Association Journal* 170:12 (June 8, 2004), pp. 1814–15; Pauline Vaillancourt Rosenau and Stephen H. Linder, "A Comparison of the Performance of For-Profit and Nonprofit U.S. Psychiatric Inpatient Care Providers since 1980," *Psychiatric Services* 54:2 (February 2003), pp. 183–87; M.J. McGregor et al., "Care Outcomes in Long-Term Care Facilities in British Columbia, Canada: Does Ownership Matter?" *Medicare Care* 44 (2006), pp. 755–68; McGregor et al., "Staffing Levels"; Kimberlyn M. McGrail et al., "For-Profit Versus Not-for-Profit Delivery of Long-Term Care," *Canadian Medical Association Journal* 176:1 (January 2, 2007), pp. 57–58.

5. André Picard, "System Shows Its Strength by Lifting Waits" *Globe and Mail*, December 20, 2005, p. A4.

6. Michael M. Rachlis, *Public Solutions to Health Care Wait Lists* (Ottawa: Canadian Centre for Policy Alternatives, 2005), p. 9.

7. Paul Krugman and Robin Wells, "The Health Care Crisis and What to Do About It," *New York Review of Books* 111:5 (March 23, 2006), p. 38.

8. Sarah Boseley, "NHS Forced to Fix Bungled Private Sector Hip Replacement Operations," *Guardian*, March 10, 2006.

9. Beth E. Jackson et al., "Gender-Based Analysis and Wait Times: New Questions, New Knowledge," a report published as an appendix to Brian D. Postl, *The Final Report of the Federal Advisor on Wait Times* (Ottawa: Health Canada, 2006).

10. Postl, *Final Report of the Federal Advisor on Wait Times*; Beth Jackson et al., "Gender-Based Analysis and Wait Times: New Questions, New Knowledge," Report 5 attached to the *Final Report of the Federal Advisor on Wait Times*.

11. See Chapter 6, note 4 for selected references on this point.

12. The provision in the 2007 federal budget making $600 million in additional transfers to the provinces in return for wait time guarantees for specific procedures within the five priority areas has attracted criticism for having scant impact. The provinces have typically taken the federal money in return for promising to meet specific targets that they were already meeting or very close to meeting. See Daniel Leblanc et al.,

"Critics Blast PM's Health Targets as 'Soft'," *Globe and Mail*, April 5, 2007, pp. A1, A4.

13. Postl, *Final Report of the Federal Advisor on Wait Times.* Arguing that a number of building blocks needed to be established to make guarantees "sustainable," Postl warned, "If you move too fast into the area of guarantees before you can actually deliver on them, you end up doing more to undermine public confidence instead of improving public confidence." Quoted in Juliet O'Neill, "Don't Rush Wait Time Guarantee," *Ottawa Citizen*, July 7, 2006. In an earlier intervention, Postl had advocated a similar, multifaceted approach to the specific issue of emergency room waits. See André Picard, "Six-Month Cure for ER Backlog Possible: Expert," *Globe and Mail*, June 29, 2000, p. A6.

14. H. Mimoto and P. Cross, "The Growth of the Federal Debt: 1975–90," *Canadian Economic Observer*, June 1991, pp. 1–17.

15. CIHI, *Health Care in Canada 2006* (Ottawa, 2006), p. 6.

16, CIHI, *Canada's Health Care Providers: 2005 Chartbook* (Ottawa, 2005), p. 43.

17. CIHI, *2005 Chartbook*, p. 43.

18. Steve Davies, *Hospital Contract Cleaning and Infection Control* (Cardiff: School of Social Science, Cardiff University, 2005) p. 31. An independent report commissioned by UNISON and available at <www.cf.ac.uk/sosci/CREST>.

19. Marcy Cohen and Marjorie Griffith Cohen, "The Politics of Pay Equity in B.C.'s Health Care System," *Canadian Woman Studies* 23:3–4 (2004), pp. 72–77. Carol Kushner, "Inside-Outside-In," slide presentation, Conference on Progressive Health Reform, Toronto, 2005.

20. Robert L. Wears and Marc Berg, "Computer Technology and Clinical Work," *Journal of the American Medical Association* 293:10 (March 9, 2005), p. 1261.

21. "Henry Mintzberg in Conversation," CBC Ideas Transcripts, Toronto, 1999, pp. 20, 22.

22. CIHI, *Health Care in Canada 2005* (Ottawa, 2005), p. 8.

23. CIHI, *Health Care in Canada 2006* (Ottawa, 2006), p. 23.

24. CBC News, "First Nurse Practitioner-Governed Clinic Opens in Sudbury," August 31, 2007 [accessed at <www.CBCNews.ca>].

25. Marcy Cohen et al., "Workload as a Determinant of Staff Injury in Intermediate Care," *International Journal of Occupational Environmental Health* 10 (2004), pp. 375–83.

26. See, for example, A. Baumann et al., *Commitment and Care: The Benefits of a Healthy Workplace for Nurses, Their Patients and the System* (Toronto: The Change Foundation and the Canadian Health Services Research Foundation, 2001).

Chapter Seven: Public Strategies and Shared Solutions

1. Calculated from *OECD Health Data 2006—Frequently Requested Data*, using Purchasing Power Parity or PPP to calculate relative spending levels without the distortions caused by international currency fluctuations. Accessed from <www.oecd.org> on September 5, 2006.

2. Robert Evans et al., "Who Are the Zombie Masters and What Do They Want?" (Toronto: Premier's Council on Health, Well-Being and Social Justice, 1994).

3. On P3 (or, as they are called in the United Kingdom, Private Finance Initiatives, or PFIs) projects, see, for example, Allyson M. Pollock et al., "Private Finance and 'Value for Money' in NHS Hospitals: A Policy in Search of a Rationale?" *British Medical Journal* 324 (May 18, 2002), pp. 1205–09; Matthew G. Dunnigan and Allyson M. Pollock, "Downsizing of Acute Inpatient Beds Associated with Private Finance Initiative: Scotland's Case Study," *British Medical Journal* 326 (April 26, 2003), pp. 905–08; Lewis Auerbach et al., *Funding Hospital Infrastructure: Why P3s Don't Work, and What Will* (Ottawa: Canadian Centre for Policy Alternatives, 2003).

4. Frank Dobson, "UK Trial with Private Health Care Is Failing," *Toronto Star*, April 12, 2007, p. A19; Jacky Davis, "As Doctors, We See the Cancer that Eats Away at the NHS," *Guardian*, June 27, 2005; John Carvel, "GPs Offered Payments to Send Patients Private," *Guardian*, May 11, 2006.

5. Cohen and Griffith Cohen, "The Politics of Pay Equity," p. 72.

6. See, for example, Jean L. Rouleau et al., "A Comparison of Management Patterns after Acute Myocardial Infarction in Canada and the United States," *New England Journal of Medicine* 328:11 (March 18, 1993); Louise Pilote et al., "Differences in the Treatment of Myocardial Infarction in the United States and Canada: Comparison of Two University Hospitals," *Archives of Internal Medicine* 154:10 (May 23, 1994); Jack V. Tu et al., "Use of Cardiac Procedures and Outcomes in Elderly Patients with Myocardial Infarction in the United States and Canada," *New England Journal of Medicine* 336:21 (May 22, 1997); Mark J. Eisenberg et al., "Outcomes and Cost of Coronary Artery Bypass Graft Surgery

in the United States and Canada," *Archives of Internal Medicine* 165 (July 11, 2005); Dennis T. Ko et al., "Quality of Care and Outcomes of Older Patients with Heart Failure Hospitalized in the United States and Canada," *Archives of Internal Medicine* 165 (November 28, 2005).

7.   Colleen Fuller, "Case Studies: Corporate Providers vs. Patients and the Public in Manitoba," *Home Care: What We Have, What We Need* (Ottawa: Canadian Health Coalition, 2001), pp. 44–50.

8.   Pat Armstrong and Tamara Daly, "Not Enough Hands," report prepared for the Canadian Union of Public Employees, 2005.

9.   CIHI, *Canada's Health Care Providers* (Ottawa, 2002), p. 87; Armstrong and Daly, "Not Enough Hands."

10. Pat Armstrong, "Closer to Home: More Work for Women," in Armstrong et al., *Take Care: Warning Signals for Canada's Health System* (Toronto: Garamond Press, 1994), pp. 95–110.

11. Decima Research, *National Profile of Family Caregivers in Canada* (Ottawa: Health Canada, 2002), p. 6.

12. K. Cranswick, "Help Close at Hand: Relocating to Give or Receive Care," *Canadian Social Trends* (Winter 1999), p. 12.

13. See the articles by Harrington, Devereaux, Rosenau and Linder, McGregor and McGrail and their colleagues, cited above in Chapter 6, note 4, for references to many of these studies.

14. Devereaux et al., "Payments for Care"; Woolhandler and Himmelstein, "High Costs"; Woolhandler et al., "Costs of Health Care Administration"; D.U. Himmelstein et al., "Who Administers? Who Cares? Medical, Administrative and Clinical Employment in the United States and Canada," *American Journal of Public Health* 86:2 (February 1996), pp. 172–88.

15. Michael Rachlis and Carol Kushner, *Strong Medicine: How to Save Canada's Health Care System* (Toronto: HarperCollins, 1994); Rachlis, *Prescription for Excellence* (Toronto: HarperCollins, 2005).

16. Krugman and Wells, "The Health Care Crisis."

17. See the *Charlottetown Declaration on the Right to Care*, available from the Canadian Women's Health Network, <www.cwhn.ca>. The set of principles elaborated in this declaration is the product of an expert consultation on home care and women's unpaid caregiving that took place in Charlottetown in 2001.

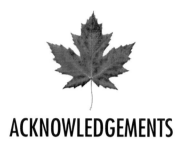

ACKNOWLEDGEMENTS

This book represents years of working with researchers, care providers, and community activists on health care issues. They all deserve credit, although we take responsibility for any errors that remain. Wayne Antony's enthusiasm for the project was infectious and his energy helped drive the book to completion. We hope it is a worthy launch for Fernwood's new series. Both Beverley Rach and Brenda Conroy were respectful and efficient in their book design and proofreading, and Robert Clarke's copy editing did much to improve the book. Pat's father once again provided the space to write in the splendid isolation of the northern woods and our daughters once again put up with our distraction. We thank them all.

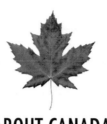

ABOUT CANADA

From health care to agriculture, child care, globalization, immigration, energy, water and more: the books in this new series will explore key issues for Canadians. About Canada books provide basic — but critical and passionate — coverage of central aspects of our society. Written in accessible language by experts in their fields, the books are presented in a popular format, at affordable prices.